Statistical Reasoning in Medicine

Springer
New York
Berlin
Heidelberg
Barcelona
Hong Kong
London
Milan
Paris
Singapore
Tokyo

Lemuel A. Moyé

Statistical Reasoning in Medicine

The Intuitive P-Value Primer

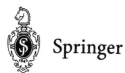 Springer

Lemuel A. Moyé
University of Texas
School of Public Health
1200 Herman Pressler
Houston, Texas 77030
USA
lmoye@utsph.sph.uth..tmc.edu

With 9 figures.

Library of Congress Cataloging-in-Publication Data
Moyé, Lemuel A.
    Statistical reasoning in medicine : the intuitive P value primer / Lemuel A. Moyé.
        p. ;   cm.
    Includes bibliographical references and index.
    ISBN 0-387-98933-1 (soft cover : alk. paper)
        1. Medicine—Research—Statistical methods.   2. Medicine—Mathematics.   3.
    Medicine—Mathematics—Miscellanea.   I. Title.
    [DNLM: 1. Statistics—methods. 2. Biometry—methods. 3. Medicine. WA 950 M938s
    2000]
    R853.S7 M698   2000
    610′.7′27—dc21   99-046511

Printed on acid-free paper.

Production managed by Jenny Wolkowicki; manufacturing supervised by Jerome Basma.
Typeset by Asco Typesetters, Hong Kong.
Printed and bound by R.R. Donnelley and Sons, Harrisonburg, VA.
Printed in the United States of America.

9 8 7 6 5 4 3 2 1

ISBN 0-387-98933-1 Springer-Verlag New York Berlin Heidelberg   SPIN 10745199

Preface

Long before I had any inkling that I would write a book, I learned that a preface is the author's attempt to engage the reader in a leisurely conversation before serious joint work begins. In that spirit, I ask you to spend a moment with me now.

Although an important focus of my training and daily work is in mathematics and statistics, I have found that many health care workers in general, and physicians in particular, have difficulty understanding research issues when they are presented mathematically. Statistical principles in medicine are relatively straightforward and can be easily absorbed without a heavy mathematical preamble. I have come to believe that the underlying research principles are not difficult; what is difficult is the mathematics in which the principles are embedded. The mathematical medium often distorts and confuses the research message for nonmathematicians. I wrote this book to explain the statistical principles in health care in fairly nonmathematical terms.

I first describe the reasoning process required to understand medical research efforts and secondly, what p values are and how to develop and interpret them. This effort is based on my experience as a physician and biostatistician both while working with colleagues at a data coordinating center for large clinical trials and in teaching courses in biostatistics to graduate students in public health. Additional impetus was provided by my work both as a statistician for the Federal Food and Drug Administration

CardioRenal Advisory Committee and as a consultant to the pharmaceutical industry.

I have regretfully concluded that, when workers in health care interpret a research effort without understanding the basic nature of statistical thinking, they grab with desperation at whatever handholds are available and unfortunately one of them is the p value. This has helped establish the view that the sweetest fruit of a research effort lies in the p value, a false perspective which is ultrareductionist, corrosive, and ultimately self-defeating. Some have called this thought evasion.[1] Since scientists and ultimately the public cannot afford to have so little understanding of these entities, I have chosen as a focal point of this book the ubiquitous p value.

Researchers have created a polluted sea of p values in which we all restlessly swim. Designed to make a simple statement about sampling error, p values have in the minds of many become the final arbiter of research efforts. Most times, at a study's inception, there is only minimal if any discussion at all of the alpha error, often relegated to the sample size computation. Commonly, the tacit assumption is that the p value at the study's end should be less than 0.05. However, during the course of the experiment's execution and conclusion, mainframe and desktop computing centers spew p values out by the tens and sometimes by the hundreds. Investigators often gnash their teeth over what this entity's value will be at the study's conclusion: <0.05 or ≥ 0.05? P values are copiously listed in many scientific manuscripts. Many researchers have turned over the decision process to the p value, conveniently and mistakenly allowing it to become the dispassionate magistrate of our labor, the final judge of the quality of our research efforts. To those workers p values are the switching signal for the research train. If the p value is less than 0.05, the research moves down the main track to manuscript publication, grant awards, regulatory approval, and academic promotion. If it is greater than 0.05, the switch moves the other way, directing the research train off to a dead-end sidetrack, into the elephants' graveyard of discarded and useless studies.

The value of p values is hotly debated. Epidemiologists have shown some signs of revolt against the p value, as the editorial policies of the *American Journal of Public Health* and *Epidemiology*

---

[1] See, for example C Poole. "Beyond the confidence interval." *American Journal of Public Health*. February 1987. Vol. 77. No 2. 195–199.

can attest. Others cling doggedly to its use. Yet, if you were to ask research physicians what a p value is and how it relates to sampling error, many would be unable to tell you. Although they have gotten the message that the p value "had better be less than oh five," they could not tell you precisely what it is that should be less than 0.05. Unfortunately, I do not think that we statisticians have been as helpful as we ought to have been. A biometry professor at a school of public health once asked a statistics student sitting for his qualifying exam (which must be passed to enter the Ph.D. candidacy phase) "Explain what a p value means." The professor never received a satisfactory response.[2] When biostatisticians do respond to this question, we often give the following response "a p value is the conditional probability of rejecting the null hypothesis in favor of the alternative hypothesis when the null hypothesis is true." I fear that, to the non-statistical world, this answer is Orwellian doublespeak.

This text is different from many books that discuss statistical inference, in the sense that it emphasizes a nonmathematical approach, teasing out the statistical reasoning from the mathematics while spending substantial time on the interpretation of significance testing. From this context, it was my purpose to produce a book that focused on the simple, basic, and ethical development, understanding, and interpretation of the p values that surround us. The solution to the p value dilemma will be supplied not by technology, but by careful deliberate reasoning. I hope this book provides a foundation for this thought process.

University of Texas   Lemuel Moyé, MD, Ph.D
School of Public Health
March 2000

---

[2] Related by Dr. Sharon Cooper.

Acknowledgments

My grandmother was half-Cherokee, and I learned much from her. One important lesson was not to begin the day, and not to stir from your bed, until you have given thanks to God for the people He has placed in your life to guide you. Good friends are His sweet encouragement. The following list cannot come close to fully acknowledging those who have supported this effort.

I owe a special debt of thanks to the leaders and members of the CardioRenal Advisory Committee to the Food and Drug Administration, on which I served as statistician from 1995 to 1999. They are Ray Lipicki, JoAnn Lindenfeld, Alastair Wood, Alexander Shepherd, Barry Massie, Cynthia L. Raehl, Michael Weber, Cindy Grimes, Udho Thadani, Robert Califf, John DiMarco, Marvin Konstam, Dan Roden and Milton Packer, I believe the public sessions held three times a year are among the best training grounds for cardiovascular research epidemiology and biostatistics. I am also in Lloyd Fisher's debt, with whom I have often disagreed and from whom I have always learned.

I am indebted to my alma mater, The University of Texas School of Public Health, and in general to public schools, which have provided much of my education. To you all, and especially to Asha Kapadia, Palmer Beasley, Robert Hardy, Charles Ford, Barry Davis, Darwin Labarthe, Richard Shekelle, Fred Annegers, and C. Morton Hawkins, consider this book an early payment on a debt too big to ever repay. Thanks to Craig Pratt and John Mahmarian, who have been patiently supportive in the development of my ideas. Also, my gratitude to Marc Pfeffer, Frank Sacks, Eugene Braunwald—you have been more influential than you know.

To the fellow classmates and friends known as the "DELTS"—Derrick Taylor, MD, Ernest Vanterpool, and Tyrone Perkins. Ever since high school in Queens, New York, we have pushed and prodded each other to excellence. Whatever I do that is worthwhile, you are part of.

I have been blessed with friends who have had a wellspring of common sense, which they have been willing to share with me. Four of them are James Powell of Cincinnati, Ohio, John McKnight of Washington D.C., Joseph Mayfield of New York, and Gilbert Ramirez of San Antonio, Texas.

Finally to Dixie, my wife, and Flora Ardon, my daughter, who are constant stars by whom I steer, and to God, who has been more faithful than I have been.

Contents

Community Expectations vs. Mandate Abrogation
Let the Investigators Decide After the Fact?
Throwing the Baby Out with the Bath Water?
    Negative Trials with Positive Secondary Endpoints
Conclusions
References

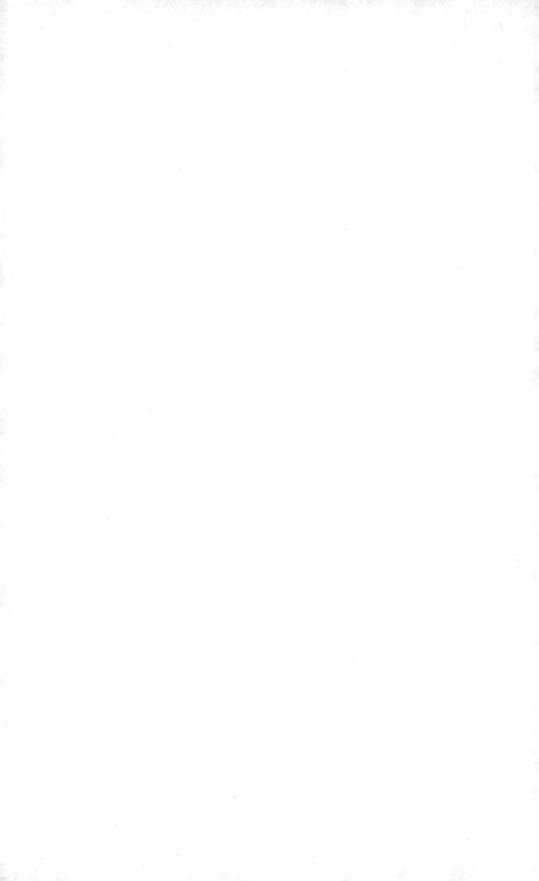

Introduction

"Dr. Moyé, will you please tell me where a p value comes from?"

It was the fall of 1977, and like every other new fourth-year medical student at Indiana University School of Medicine, I was thinking hard about life after medical school. With an undergraduate degree in applied mathematics, I had decided to go to graduate school in statistics after I became a physician. However, several practicing doctors had convinced me that it would be best if I first obtained a license to practice medicine, and the most accepted way of doing that was to complete an internship. My personal life at the time required that I stay in Indianapolis for any post-medical school work, so, while my classmates applied to many hospitals across the country (and sometimes around the world), I applied to only two, and was interested in only one— Methodist Hospital Graduate Medical Center. After completing the required forms, I received in the mail an acknowledgement of my application and a schedule of interviews with physicians at Methodist Hospital. Prominent on the list was Dr. William Kassell, Chairman of Obstetrics and Gynecology.

Obstetrics and Gynecology had been my first clinical rotation after psychiatry as a junior, and, like most third-year students, I fumbled mightily with the new clinical learning curve, often studying many hours to gain one hour's worth of knowledge. Therefore, I was surprised to see, upon applying for my internship that my exposure to this specialty was not over yet. Dr. Kassell was known as the tough-minded, practical chairman of the prestigious Obstetrics and Gynecology Department of Methodist Hospital. Like most good chiefs, he mixed fairness and high expectations.

The night before the interview was memorable for its self-inflicted brutality. I dragged out my old notes in OB-GYN, reviewing relations between colposcopy findings and cervical cancer treatment procedures. I memorized again the workup of pre-eclampsia. By morning, my brain was jammed full of obstetrical information.

Now I was in Dr. Kassell's office, and seemed to watch from afar as he gruffly mumbled a greeting my way and waved me to sit in a chair facing him over his expansive desk, heaped high with textbooks, papers, and hospital charts. I awaited the one question for which I had not prepared the night before—the one question that would send my plans crashing. It came forth in a gasp of exasperation from the great man: "Dr. Moyé, will you please tell me where a p value comes from?"

I was stunned! However, the question was real and I had to give an answer. It turns out that, just prior to my interview, the chairman had reviewed a manuscript for his journal club (the author and topic I have long since forgotten). P values had played a prominent role in this manuscript and were apparently being used as the yardstick against which the results were measured. It seemed to him as if these p values were like some great, final, unfeeling arbiter of positive or negative results. Dr. Kassell had reviewed my record and, seeing my undergraduate background in statistics, thought he would spend our interview time discussing this research issue.

This book is for everyone, regardless of their current position, one who has asked (or has wanted to ask) Dr. Kassell's question and wanted a comprehensible, nonmathematical answer. *Statistical Reasoning in Medicine: The Intuitive P Value Primer* focuses on first the underlying principles of statistical thought in medicine and secondly, the ethical development and interpretation of p values in health care research. It is written for workers in health care who have to interpret statistics in medical research. A physician confronted with a new finding in his or her field, a director in a pharmaceutical company attempting to draw the correct conclusion from a series of experiments on a promising new product, an authority who sits on an advisory panel for the government and decides whether to advise the government to approve a product all must have an understanding of p values and the underlying statistical thinking. If you are a decision maker and do not have in-depth training in statistics, but now find that, in order to make the best decision possible, you must grapple with the thorny theory of statistical reasoning and the slippery issue of p values, then this book is for you.

With an emphasis on patient and community protection, *The P Value Primer* develops and emphasizes the p value concept while deemphasizing the mathematics, providing examples of the p value's correct implementation and interpretation in a manner consistent with the preeminent principle of clinical research programs: "First, do no harm". In addition to being an overview of p value utilization, this book breaks new ground with the creation of type I error bounds that are nontraditional, innovative, easy to use, and consistent with both the patient protective and and community protective ethics of health care researchers.

The *P Value Primer* begins with a description of the controversies that have engulfed statistical reasoning for four hundred years, providing a brief history of statistical inference and how p values got their start (prologue). The requirement of sample based research is developed from first principles, building up the reader's nonmathematical intuition of the notion of sampling error, culminating in a useful definition of p values in laymen's terms. Starting with simple problems in p value interpretation, this book moves on to describe the correct use of p values in health research. The natural, intuitive, and nonmathematical notion of study concordance (where an experiment analysis plan is immune to incoming data) vs. study discordance (where the analysis plan itself is severely affected by the data) is introduced and used as the basis for deciding if p value interpretation should proceed (chapter 1).

Progressing from there, the problems with using the traditional p value threshold of 0.05 are explicitly discussed (chapter 2). The difficulty of p value interpretation in epidemiological studies is covered in detail (chapter 3), and the differences between p values and effect sizes is emphasized (chapter 4). The notion of power and sample size computation is developed from first principles for the reader (chapter 5). From there, we begin to discuss in nonmathematical terms some deeper issues in alpha allocation and p value interpretation, beginning with ethical justification for asymmetric apportionment of alpha (chapter 6). I then describe new alpha allocation procedures that should be used in experiments with multiple clinical endpoints, recently introduced into the peer-reviewed literature (chapters 7 and 8). P value interpretation in regression analysis is covered (chapter 9), and the development of p values from the Bayes approach is discussed (chapter 10). Finally, discussions of the difficulties of subgroup analyses and data dredging are provided, with the focus remaining on p value interpretation (chapter 11). The book ends with a conclusion, providing concrete advice to the reader for experimental design and p value construction, offering specifics on when the p values of others should be ignored.

The unique feature of *The P Value Primer* is its nonmathematical concentration on the underlying statistical reasoning process in clinical research. I have come to believe that this focus is sorely lacking and greatly missed in standard statistical textbooks that emphasize the details of test statistic construction and computational tools. We will consciously deemphasize computational devices (e.g., paired t testing, the analysis of variance, and Cox regression analysis), focusing instead on the features of experimental design that either clarify or blur p value interpretation. This book recognizes that there will be inevitable tension between the mathematics of significance testing and the ethical requirements in medical research, and concentrates on the resolution of these issues in p value interpretation. Furthermore, the omnipresent concern for ethics is a consistent tone of this book. In this day and age of complicated clinical experiments, in which new medications can inflict debilitating side effects on patients and their families, and where experiments have multiple clinical measures of success, we will provide concrete, clear advice on the construction of alpha errors, using easily understood computations, e.g., the asymmetric apportionment of alpha and the intelligent allocation of alpha among a number of primary and secondary endpoints in clinical experiments.

The P Value *Primer* is written at a level requiring only one introductory course in applied statistics as a prerequisite, putting its concepts well within reach of any health care worker who has had a brief health statistics background. It will be valuable to physicians, research nurses, health care researchers, program directors in the pharmaceutical industry, and government workers in the food or drug regulatory industry who must critique research results. It would also be useful as an additional text for graduate students in public health programs, medical and dental students, and students in the biological sciences.

That's all fine, but how did I answer Dr. Kassell back in 1977? Fortunately, I answered him accurately, but unfortunately, I answered him (from the viewpoint of many) unintelligibly. I am sure that I gave the knee-jerk response many statisticians give, i.e., "A p value is the conditional probability of rejecting the null hypothesis when the null hypothesis is true". However, even though this answer is technically correct, I could never shake the feeling that, after hearing this terse, reflexive reply, the listener remains befuddled about what these p values really are, and why they have become so important. Like the newcomer to a foreign language who gets a verbose reply to a short, hesitant question, the inquisitor is satisfied that the answer is somewhere in there but has no clue exactly what the answer is.

Unfortunately, too many listeners have gotten the message that whatever they are, p values had better be "less than 0.05" before the results of the research program can be labeled "significant." Since significance is often converted into manuscript publication, grant awards, or regulatory approval, the sense is that "you better be less than oh five or they won't accept you." We will take some time to push a little beyond that traditional notion as well.

Prologue: "Let Others Thrash it out!" A Brief History

The Arabic doctor Avicenna in the eleventh century provided seven rules for medical experimentation involving human subjects [1]. Among these precepts was a recommendation for the use of control groups, the advice of repeating results (replication), and a warning against the use of variables that would confuse Avidenna's decision about what variable is actually causing the effect of interest. These observations represented a great intellectual step forward; however, this step was taken in relative isolation. An additional six hundred years had to pass before the line of reasoning that led to p values eventually emerged. In order to understand the initial twists and turns of the development of this curious discipline, we need to take a quick diversion to life in Europe five hundred years ago.

Europe's emergence from the Middle Ages

Insuring society's survival before developing society's statistics was the necessary order of progress and, in the 1500s, Europe was still struggling with its uneven emergence from the provincialism and ignorance of the Middle Ages. Groups of people were beginning to come together in greater numbers. Altogether, Europe

1

had at least twenty cities in twelve countries with populations over one hundred thousand, including Naples, Lisbon, Moscow, St. Petersburg, Vienna, Amsterdam, Berlin, Rome, and Madrid. The biggest cities in Europe were London and Paris [2]. This movement to urbanization slowly accelerated creating new links of interdependence among the new city dwellers. However, with little knowledge about themselves, these cities remained blind to their own needs, and had no control over their social progress.

Although rural inhabitants vastly outnumbered urban dwellers, the contrasts between a large city with its education and culture and the surrounding, often poverty-stricken, countryside were striking. Towns lived off the countryside not by buying produce, but by using tithes, rents, and dues to acquire rural products from peasants, widening the disparity of wealth. For example, the residents of Palermo in Sicily consumed one-third the island's food production while paying only one-tenth of the taxes [2]. Peasants often resented the prosperity of towns and their exploitation of the countryside to serve urban interests.

However, cities had their own share of problems. Despite an end to the most devastating ravages of plague, cities still experienced high death rates (especially among children) because of unsanitary living conditions, polluted water, and a lack of sewage facilities. One observer compared the stench of Hamburg to an open sewer that could be smelled for miles around. Overcrowding became a problem as cities continued to grow from an influx of rural immigrants looking for work. Unfortunately, cities proved no paradise for these unskilled workers, who found few employment opportunities awaiting them. The result was a serious problem of poverty in the eighteenth century [2]. Why was this intolerable situation tolerated? One reason was that there was no quantitation of these problems—each citizen had his or her own experience, but there was no person or group which had a corporate sense of the quality of life. The only standard for the current quality of life was rural life, and this, everyone agreed was worse than the current urban conditions. In realizing only that they were better off in the city than in the countryside, these denizens did not have the time or leisure to wonder whether their own lives in the city could be improved. It was commonly accepted that living condition improvement occurred slowly over centuries—not within a lifetime. This was far too slow a progression to try to keep track of or to influence.

However, no one could avoid the great issue of urban poverty.

Poverty was a highly visible problem in the eighteenth century both in cities and in the countryside.[1] It has been estimated that in France and Britain ten percent of the people were dependent on charity or begging for food. Earlier in Europe the poor had been viewed as blessed children of God, and the duty of Christians was to assist them. However, there soon began a change to a less charitable attitude toward the impoverished, the newer perspective suggesting that the poor were best viewed as slovenly and unwilling to work themselves out of their lot. In this growing cauldron of social conflict began a furvor for change, and the need to understand these huge new collections of humanity. Since the cities were certainly made up of individuals, were there not some features of the whole urban unit that could be influenced? With no place to turn, urban dwellers looked to the ruling classes.

The ruling class was the power center, and, everywhere in Europe class privileges and the old order remained strong. Unfortunately, the monarchs had no interest in comprehending their subjects—only in taxing them. Taxes were the means by which the monarchs made war, and by knowing the total number of citizens, these rulers could better estimate how much revenue could be raised. Leaders sought to enlarge not their understanding, but their tax collection bureaucracies in order to raise revenue to support the new large standing armies. Thus, the first issues in statistics were issues not of statistical hypothesis testing, but of simple counting—the basis of demography.

These early demographers had a daunting task, for there was no reliable data on which to base populations size claims, and anything approximating modern census machinery was nonexistent. Clearly, the idea of a census was well known, having being described in the New Testament[3]. However, there were two obstacles to its development and use in eighteenth century England. The first was the understandable unwillingness of the population to participate, as they feared that their involvement would lead either directly or indirectly to higher taxes. The second was the tendency of the government to keep what poorly inaccurate de-

[1] In Venice, licensed beggars made up 3 to 5 percent of the population while unlicensed beggars may have constituted as much as 13 to 15 percent. Beggars in Bologna, Italy, were estimated at 25 percent of the population while figures indicate that, in Mainz, Germany, 30 percent of the people were beggars or prostitutes [2].

mographic data it did have a secret, because of its possible military value. The ingenuity of early demographers was tested as they worked to obtain indirect estimates of the population's size, age and sex distribution. Multiplying the number of chimneys by an assumed average family size, or inferring age distribution from registered information concerning time of death were typical enumeration procedure [4].

Nevertheless, taxes were collected, which guaranteed the existence of armies, which guaranteed wars [2]—and the wars were brutal. The involvement of five great powers, including France and Britain, in conflict from the Far East to the New World, (the Seven Years' War) initiated a new scale of conflict that could legitimately be viewed as the first world war. Everywhere in Europe, the increased demands for taxes to support these large, terrible conflicts, with no coincident desire to learn about (as a first step in providing for) these taxed populations, fueled cries for change. Virulent diatribes on the privileged orders, caught the ruling monarchs unprepared. This social ferment, in coincidence with sustained population growth, dramatic changes in finance, trade, and industry, and the growth of poverty created tensions that undermined the foundations of the old order [2].

Thus use of early data tabulations was restricted to adding to the burdens of the population, and not used for alleviating their suffering. This indirectly led to demands for tax relief and calls for a restructured social order. The monarchs' inability to deal meaningfully with these stipulations led to a revolutionary outburst at the end of the eighteenth century heralding the beginning of the end of absolute royal law. When the tension became to great, the monarchs gave way and the people turned away from them to the new forces in their lives, introduced by the Industrial Revolution. Attention to the old order was replaced by attention to technology and profit.

Intellectual Triumph: The Industrial Revolution

The Industrial Revolution, recognized as a great turning point in human history, began to transform culture from the inside out, as muscle power (human and animal) was replaced by other forms of energy. The Industrial Revolution was a triumph of that intellect. Unlike the ethereal forces which directed peoples' loyalties to the old order of monarchies, the Industrial Revolution required quantitative knowledge in ever-increasing amounts, and had the advantage of a direct and sometimes immediate improvement in one's well-being. Not a onetime jump in productivity and wealth, this revolution began a process of ever-accelerating change.

Of all European countries, England was the best poised for this propulsive movement forward.[2] Because of low interest rates and the presence of a stable government, money was cheap, taxes were low, and traditional restrictions on enterprise (such as guilds) had been substantially weakened. The result was a cascade of innovation as one invention sparked another. The development of the flying shuttle, the spinning jenny, the water frame, the power loom, and the spinning mule in the eighteenth century were just a few of the technical innovations that appeared, increasing product output. Furthermore, iron and steel production made large-scale mechanization possible. A relatively well-fed workforce used these technologies for achieving unanticipated new levels of productivity. The fruits of their productive efforts could be either sold at home or easily shipped abroad. During this process the driving social question changed from "Will I survive" to "How can I prosper". The issue of survival began to change to the issue of quality of life. Although there were as yet no demographic measures of this quality, there arose a collective sense that it could and must be raised.

Therefore, an immediate benefit of the Industrial Revolution activity was pressure for the occurrence of and resultant higher standard of living in the 1700s. New, larger markets led to improved transportation systems.[3] New agricultural techniques decreased the vulnerability of food crops to bad weather. There were improvements in fodder crops, with a subsequent rise in

---

[2] While the great European conflagrations in the fifteenth through seventeenth centuries changed little on the European continent, victories brought the emergence of Great Britain as the world's greatest naval and colonial power. Great Britain had the best combination of resources, access to markets, and institutions. As an island, England was secure from invasion and more open to overseas markets. Property owners had an important role in the English government and therefore not need to fear it as their interest in industrial development and profit increased.

[3] In France, the time it took for a road trip from Paris to Marseilles dropped from 12 days to 8 between 1765 and 1780.

meat production, in England. Coal was used as fuel. The new use of fire-resistant materials (brick and tile) produced by coal heat led to a drop in the number of disastrous fires in cities and a consequent conservation of resources needed for rebuilding. A new belief in the principle of wastage avoidance paralleled the development of both insurance and government-sponsored stockpiling of food surplus. Quarantine measures helped to eliminate the plague after 1720. The population of London increased from 20,000 in the year 1500 to 500,000 by 1700. People became healthier, stronger, better-rested, and more comfortable and looking anew at their surroundings, began to wonder what the true limits to growth really were.

Intellectual activity was thriving, and the spirit of enterprise was respectable. Many prosperous people were involved in productive economic activity. As opposed to the closely guarded estimates of population size, technical know-how in the marketplace and the incipient halls of science was not restricted to a few geniuses, but shared by many. Artists, e.g. Turner and the Impressionists were inspired and excited by the new industries. Likewise the productive climate and the improved standard of living made intellectual initiative respectable. This was a time when old facts long accepted without proof were unceremoniously discarded by men who themselves would answer questions by querying nature directly without appealing to monarchs. However, even the most basic information on the citizenry of England itself was nonexistent.

The Rise of Political Arithmetic

With the improved standard of living, new information about the English, for the English, was required. Was the population growing or shrinking (Some believed at the time that the population of London was over two million, an exorbitant estimate.) The rise of capitalism required estimates of the demographics of the population, and, of course, the monarchs were still interested in taxation.

The first major contribution to early demography was by John Graunt, who published "Natural History and Political Observations on the London Bills of Mortality". His work led to the establishment of the universal registration of births and marriages, not for religious purposes, but for the purposes of accurate reports to the government. He provided some unique computations by counting burials to estimate the proportion of deaths. From this preliminary work, Graunt showed that the estimates of one million or even two million citizens living in London, which were being blithely used as population size estimates were completely inaccurate. He was the first to realize the importance not just of collecting basic demographic data, but of studying these "vital statistics." William Petty received impetus from Graunt's early tabulations, and together they labored together to develop the first life table, allowing a crude estimate of death rates in London. Under their auspices, information was collected on the number of deaths and causes of death, leading to the first scientifically based estimates of cause-specific death rates. For the first time, the ravishes of bubonic plague were categorized, as well as the number of deaths from consumption and "phthisis" (tuberculosis) [5].

However illuminating these first demographic investigations were, the innovative workers behind them were not known as "statisticians"; that particular term was applied to an unrelated field. The term "statisticus" was derived from the Italian "statistica" meaning "statesman." The term was first used by Gottfried A. Achenwall in 1752 to describe a branch of knowledge that we would describe today as constitutional history [5]. In the eighteenth century a statistician did not collect data, and had nothing to do with mathematics; statisticians were seen as academicians who cerebrated about "the state." Early works in statistics were not data oriented or mathematical at all; they were theses in political science. The contemporary term for the infant demography work of Graunt and Perry in the early 1700s was "political arithmetic" [5].

The Role of Religion in Political Arithmetic

It is evident that the collection of this first vital statistics data by Graunt and Perry ignited an explosion of questions, not all of them scientific. Although the work started as simple tabulations of the total number of people in London, and gender distribution, other more interesting questions rapidly followed: "Why are there more burials than christenings? How many men are married? How many are fighting men? How long does it take to replenish housing after a wave of the plague? How many men ignore their civic duties? In what proportion do men neglect the orders of the church?" These were in turn followed by hotly debated answers. The fiery issue of interpretation of statistical data in a religiously charged and politically polarized environment ignited at once in England.

It is impossible to understand the world of seventeenth-eighteenth century England without paying explicit attention to the overwhelming issue of religion [6]. Religion was seen at the time not just as a private matter, but as the vital, sustaining bond that held society together, serving as the foundation of all forms of political organization. Religion permeated all respectable lives, playing a prominent role in public commerce, and collisions between religious ideas were matters of central importance to English life. Therefore new questions whose answers charac-terized the spiritual state of the English and led to broad, new de-scriptors of the urban population had instant religious overtones. The clerics themselves stood disunited on the important religious issues of the day, being themselves involved in bitter internecine disputes. In the sixteenth century, the general struggle between the Roman Catholics and the "Reformed" or Protestant churches had been resolved on the basis of a compromise under the Tudors. The settlement held that the monarch would be the head of a national Anglican church which was part Catholic (High Church) and part Protestant (Low Church) in structure, doctrine, and dogma. However, this shared power was shattered with the ac-cession of Queen Elizabeth I to the throne of England in 1558, marking the decisive victory of Protestantism as the supremacy of the Pope was rejected [6].

However, the recently formed Protestant leadership unraveled as utterances of the word "Puritan" began. This new sect within the Protestants' own councils held that the work of Protestant ref-ormation was not made complete by the repudiation of the Pope's teachings. By the middle of the seventeenth century the Puritans were a large and broad ranging group in English society. Serious and intelligent, Puritans wielded profound influence within the local communities. This sect, with its strong patriotism and fierce anti-Catholic creed became a force to be reckoned with in trade and commerce. Puritans were also influential among the aristoc-racy, larger landowners, and lawyers who made up the membership of the Houses of Parliament. Thus, their influence extended throughout English society, from the local neighborhoods up to and including national office. By this time, however, even the Puritans were divided amongst themselves on matters of church organization.

This contentious relationship between Catholics, non-Puritan Protestants, and Puritans was directly translated to the political arena. All intellectual work was interpreted in this religiously charged, polarized environment, with the competing philosophies spilling over into contentious interpretations of the early demographers' work. Even John Graunt's reputation was besmirched by his conversion to Catholicism late in life. Graunt's work was criticized, and he himself sustained vilification, finally being subjected to the outrageous accusation that he was responsible for the great fire of London [5]. We nod with ironic appreciation as we see that these early demographers were called not statisticians, but political arithmeticians.

"Let Others Thrash It Out!"

This description of demography as political arithmetic lasted for approximately one hundred years. In 1798, the Scotsman Sir John Sinclair applied the word "statistics" to the data and methods of political arithmetic. This led to a bitter turf war over who would be called a statistician (the political scientists or the data tabulators), especially in Germany, where the political science use of the word, "statistics" really took root [5]. However, in the end, statistics took on its mathematical, data-oriented meaning and the older idea of "statistics" moving to the areas of political economy, political science, and constitutional law and history. Throughout this period, the demographers' technical problem of estimation was taken up by the mathematicians Halley and DeMoivre, spreading to Bernoulli, Euler, and other mathematicians throughout Europe. They expanded into the works of Poisson and Laplace, which became the foundation of the laws of probability and the inception of the mathematical science of statistics.

However, the issue of statistical inference proved to be tougher, taking an interesting turn in 1830 when a proposal was made to form a statistics section of the British Association for the Advancement of Science. Under the august leadership of Thomas Malthus, a subcommittee was created to answer the question, "Is statistics a branch of science? The committee readily agreed that insofar as statistics dealt with the collection and orderly tabulation of data; that indeed was science. However on the question "Is the statistical interpretation of the results scientifically respectable?", a violent split arose between those who wanted to include the inferential aspect of statistics and those who stood against inference. The anti-inference sect won out, repeating their victory a few years later in 1834 when the Statistical Society of London (later to become the Royal Statistical Society) was formed. Their victory was symbolized in the emblem chosen by the Society. This was a fat, neatly bound sheaf of healthy wheat—presumably representing the abundant data collected and neatly tabulated. On the binding ribbon was the Society's motto—*Aliis exterendum*, which means "Let others thrash it out" [7].

What a curious decision! A contributing factor could have been that many of the senior statisticians of the time were heads of official statistical agencies, whose tasks were confined to the collection and tabulation of data. Interpreters of data bearing on social, economic, or political matters often disagreed violently as to the conclusions drawn from the data, a conflict that we recognize continues to this day. However, by 1840, the Society began to push hard against this limitation.

Early Experimental Design

Although the political arithmeticians worked in urban environments, much of the development of comparative experimentation was carried out in agricultural field experimentation in the eighteenth and nineteenth centuries. Developments in experimental design paralleled but were set apart from the development of probability. This work in agricultural science was fundamentally different from the work of Graunt and Petty, because experimental design is not a matter of tabulation but of controlling the application of an intervention (e.g. new seed). It remains a curiosity that the development of experimental methodology could proceed without the direct involvement of the early probabilists. Perhaps this is reflective of the degree to which the powers of observation and deductive reasoning could be strengthened without heavy reliance on mathematics.

In 1627, Francis Bacon published an account of the effects of steeping wheat seeds in nine different "nutrient mixtures" on germination speed and the heartiness of growth[4] [7]. In the eighteenth century, a body of useful contributions to experimental design was constructed by a relatively unknown experimentalist. In 1763, a young man, Arthur Young, inherited a farm in England. Only eight years later, he had carried out a large number of field experiments and published his conclusions in a three-volume book, *A Course of Experimental Agriculture* (1771). His insight was clear, and he developed ideas easily recognized as fundamental to experimental methodology. For example, Young stressed that experiments must be comparative, insisting that, when comparing a new method and standard method, both must be present in the experiment [9][5].

Young also recognized that even in comparative experiments, many factors other then the intervention being tested in the experiment influenced the outcome of the experiment. Soil fertility, drainage, and insects, among other factors, all contributed to increasing or decreasing yields in each of the experimental plots. Because the sum effect of them affecting plot yields in different ways, some years increasing the yield, and in some years decreasing it, the results of a single experiment in one year could not be completely trusted. Thus, Young concluded that since each trial was subject to these influences, he therefore often replicated his experiments five times (once a year or once a growing season)[9]. This was a first attempt to come to grips with the notion of variability in experiments results. His solution of replication is one that is commonly and of necessity invoked today. Young also stressed careful measurements. When it was time to determine the experiment's outcome, all his expenses that could be traced to the intervention being tested were recorded in pounds, shillings, pence, halfpennies, and farthings [9]. At harvest one sample of wheat from each of the control field and the treatment field was sent to market on the same day to determine the selling price.

These important principles of experimental design (control, reproducibility, and precision) do not at first glance have anything to do with probability; they have more to do with clarity of observation and the ability to attribute an effect to an intervention. Although Young had no quantitative technique for statistical analy-

---

[4] He determined that wine was not helpful, but that urine was [8].
[5] An early warning against the use of historical controls.

sis, he was remarkably aware of two problems that are very relevant today. One is the problem of the non-objectivity of the investigator. Each of his books begins with what is recognizable as a literature review, with examples of how some authors slant the presented data to support their favored conclusion. Furthermore, Young was well aware of the mistake of drawing conclusions that extend beyond the experimental results to the broader set of circumstances to which we want to apply the experimental results, i.e., the dangers of experimental extrapolation. He warned that his own conclusions about the influences of crop development and growth could not be trusted to apply to a different farm with different soil and land management practices. By carefully noting that his results would not apply as a guide to long-term agricultural policy, he stressed the pitfalls of what we now call extrapolation and inference from a sample to a population [9].

Seventy-eight years later, James Johnson followed with the book *"Experimental Agriculture"* (1849), a treatise devoted to practical advice on experimental design [7]. Johnson stressed the importance of doing experiments well. A badly conceived experiment, he said, was not merely a waste of time and money but, had much broader implications. It led to the incorporation of incorrect results into standard books. It also led to the loss of money, as other farmers attempted to follow its precepts, and to the neglect of further researchers. This seminal work also reflected Johnson's careful experimental observations. He observed that plots of land near one another tended to give similar yields. Hence he recommended that repetitions of the same treatment be spread across noncontiguous plots[6]. The consequence of this placement was the balancing of the common soil effect throughout the control and experimental plots of the experiment. Building on Young's work, Johnson recognized the potentially destabilizing influence of soil fertility, and attempted to deal with its variability by plot distribution. This presaged the use of randomization as a technique for balancing these influences. Johnson realized, however, that his own treatment scattering maneuver to reduce the influence of variation was not enough, thereby recognizing his unfulfilled requirement for a quantitative theory of variation. [7]

---

[6] This was carried out by placing repetitions of the same treatment in relation to one another by the knight's move in chess.

Fisher, Student, and the Modern Era of Experimental Design

Born in East Finchley, London in 1890, Ronald Aylmer Fisher grew to be one of the giants in epidemiological thinking. Obtaining his schooling at Gonville and Caius College, in Cambridge, he started work in 1919 as a statistician at Rothamsted Experimental Station. He rapidly developed an interest in designing and analyzing agricultural experiments [7]. However, he realized, as Johnson had, that better methods were necessary to consider the natural variability of crop yields.

A major step forward in the theory of measuring effects in the presence of random variation had been taken while Fisher was still in training, the result appearing in the 1908 manuscript "The probability error of a mean" [10]. Its author was William D. Gosset, using the pseudonym "Student." On leaving Oxford, Gosset went to work in 1899 as a Brewer in Dublin for Guinness, a brewery whose owners preferred that their employees use pen names in their published papers[7]. Gosset's work there exposed him to many measurement problems where estimation was required from small samples. He was well aware of the problems of obtaining estimates from small samples of data, which had concerned Galton, another statistician—there just weren't enough observations in the sample to get a good sense for the distribution of the data. To estimate the variance in small samples was also difficult, for the same reason.

Gosset began by choosing the normal distribution for simplicity, stating "It appears probable that the deviation from normality must be severe to lead to serious error" [10]. He then showed that the sample mean and sample standard deviations from a normal distribution were uncorrelated and he correctly deduced that they were independent. The finding of independence simplified his next tasks immensely, leading to the identification of the distribution of the ratio $(x - \bar{x})/s$ as a t distribution (now known as Student's t distribution). Thus, experimentalists could now identify the distribution of this normed difference even when the

---

[7] This requirement of a brewery that its employees use pen names when publishing always seemed odd to me. Apparently, the Guinnes Brewery had given permission for the publication of the first scientific paper by one its employees on the condition that a pseudonym be used, possibly because competing companies might become knowledgable about ongoing work at Guinness [1, 11].

small sample size precluded a precise measure of the population variance. Agricultural scientists like Fisher could now incorporate the variance of the plot yield into a measure of the difference in plot yields and find the distribution of this normed difference, identifying extreme values.

Fisher's earliest writing on the general strategy in field experimentation appeared in the first edition of his book *Statistical Methods for Research Workers* (1925) [12], and in a short paper in 1926 "The arrangement of field experiments" [13]. This brief paper contained many of the principal ideas on the planning of experiments, including the idea of significance testing. It is in this paper that the notion of a 5 percent level of significance first appears. Since this notion has become so deeply rooted in statistical thinking, I have elaborated some upon the case that generated this concept.

The example Fisher used to demonstrate his reasoning for significance testing was an assessment of the influence of manure on crop yield. Two neighboring acres of land were to be used in a study. The first was treated with manure; the second was left without manure but was otherwise treated the same. Crops were planted and, upon harvest, the results were evaluated. The yield on the manure-treated acre was 10 percent higher than that of the non-manured acre. Although this suggested a benefit attributable to the manure, Fisher grappled with how one could decide that the greater yield was due to the manure and not just to the random play of chance. He focused on the likelihood that the yield would be 10 percent greater with no manure (i.e., without any differences between the plots). The differences between the yields of plots which were themselves treated the same was termed sampling variability. Fisher began by noting that if the sampling variability did not produce a 10 percent difference in crop yield, then

"... the evidence would have reached a point which may be called the verge of significance; for it is convenient to draw the line at about the level at which we can say 'Either there is something in the treatment or a coincidence has occurred such as does not occur more than once in twenty trials.' This level, which we may call the 5 per cent level point, would be indicated, though very roughly, by the greatest chance deviation observed in twenty successive trials." [13].

This appears to be the first mention of the 5 percent level of significance. Note that the underlying philosophy is rooted in the notion of what might have been expected to occur naturally, i.e., under the influence of only random variation. The use of the occurrence of naturally occurring events as a surrogate for random variability is remarkably similar to the thinking of the eighteenth century physician, Dr. John Arbuthnot. In 1710 he was concerned about the tendency for there to be more male births than female births registered in London [14] in each of eighty-two successive years. He understood that this tendency might be due to chance alone, and not due to some other influence. If it was due to chance alone, the probability of this event should be relatively high. He therefore computed the probability that in each of 82 successive years there were more male than female births by chance. This event had a very small probability, $(\frac{1}{2}^{82})$. He interpreted this probability as strong evidence against this event occurring by chance, and decided that there was some other systematic influence driving the relatively high number of male births. This was perhaps the earliest use of a formal probability calculation for a purpose in statistical inference [15]. Fisher went on, adding

> "If one in twenty does not seem high enough odds, we may, if we prefer it, draw the line at one in fifty (the 2 per cent point) or one in a hundred (the 1 per cent point). Personally, the writer prefers to set the low standard of significance at the 5 per cent point, and ignore entirely all results which fail to reach this level) ". [13]

The significance level of 0.05 was born from these rather casual remarks [7]. It cannot be emphasized enough that there is no deep mathematical theory that points to 0.05 as the optimum type I error level. Fisher also developed the notion of the use of randomization of the intervention in the agricultural experiment, the factorial design (analysis of variance), and the role of hypothesis testing.

We accept this thinking as the mantra of experimental design today, but these were radical concepts seventy years ago, sharply contested and heatedly debated. Published papers by Berkson [15–16] and Fisher [17] provide some feel for the technical repartee exchanged between researchers as they struggled to understand all of the implications of the hypothesis testing scenarios. Joseph Berkson was especially critical. He felt that Karl Pearson's maxim of "After all, the higher statistics are only common sense reduced to numerical appreciation" was violated by Fisher's seemingly reverse-logic significance testing arguments. Much of the criticism he leveled at Fisher was in the interpretation of the extreme findings (i.e., levels of significance) from the data. Returning to Fisher's manure example at the five percent level, just because the 10 percent yield produced on the field treated with manure would not be anticipated in twenty experiments does not preclude its occurrence by chance. Berkson argued that, if we accept the notion that it is relatively rare for a human who is between twenty and thirty years of age to die, a statistician would conclude, confronted with a dead person in his twenties, that the dead person was not human! This was amusingly refuted (although the refutation was not always amusingly received) by Fisher, who said that "It is not my purpose to make Dr. Berkson seem ridiculous nor of course for me to prevent him from providing innocent entertainment" [17]. The difficulty was that many workers were looking for arguments of certainty, while all Fisher could provide was an assessment of likelihood.

Gradually and often grudgingly, the notion of hypothesis testing began to take root in other scientific disciplines. However, some statisticians, feeling constrained by the limitations of hypothesis testing and its enforcement of a conclusion about a data set's interpretation, have pushed for more than significance testing. Rather than draw a conclusion about the value of a parameter from its sample estimate (e.g., the value of the population mean μ from the value of the sample mean), they have argued that the data may provide support for more than one value of μ. These workers have advocated that a graph of the likelihood function (the product of the probability distributions that derived from the sample of independent observations) would display the data's support for different values of μ. Some have gone so far as to suggest that reports of experimental results in scientific journals should be descriptions of likelihood functions when adequate mathematical-statistical models, can be assumed rather than just reports of significance levels or confidence interval estimates [15]. This elaborate perspective was forcefully challenged as representing patently bad advice. Jerome Cornfield believed that any scientist who attempted to publish based on a result presentation featuring an abstract likelihood function would not be published, the graphs being unintelligible [15]. Thus, although the likelihood function may be desirable, it would be unsatisfactory for scientific reporting. Cornfield further said that the early realization of its lack of utility in publications led Fisher and other statisticians to reject the likelihood function presentation in favor of significance testing and confidence intervals.

The technique of significance testing itself was to undergo a refinement into its present form. At its inception, the report of the hypothesis testing was more closely linked to the alpha level specified at the trial's inception before any data was collected. For example, if it was decided during the design phase of the experiment that the maximum value of the type I error was 0.05, the final results were reported as only $p < 0.05$ — the exact value was not computed. However, as the use of significance testing grew, there began a growing belief that this estimate of the level of significance should be sharpened. Thus, it became the custom to report the exact p value ($p = 0.021$) and not just the inequality ($p < 0.05$). This is what is carried out today.

Conclusions

Although statistics has been a recognized science for 250 years, the role of statisticians in drawing conclusions from data is still a source of contention. As recently as 1986, a spirited debate on the usefulness of p values ignited in the public health literature [19–26]. There has been a recent statement that a major epidemiological journal discourages the use of p values [27]. The idea of a p value broke into the mainstream of scientific reasoning from the confines of agricultural experiments and, although some have argued that it is a concept of exclusion and negation rather than one of inclusion and affirmation, the paradigm slowly gained acceptance even though criticism of its principles and decision rules have not yet abated. Fisher argued that research results with a p value greater than 0.05 should clearly be ignored. Although this decision was defensible for one experiment with two treatments and one endpoint, recent complexities in experimental design have required that this notion be stretched and adapted, perhaps to the breaking point. Nevertheless, the role of p values has been continually debated from their earliest inception to the present day. Never completely accepted by the entire scientific community, they are commonly used and commonly misinterpreted.

References

1. Gehan, E. and Lemak, N.A., (1994) *Statistics in Medical Research,* Plenum Medical Book Company, New York.
2. Rempel, G., (Germany Lectures). Western New England College.
3. Luke 2:1, Holy Bible. (1978) New International Version. Zondervan Bible Publishers, Grand Rapids, MI.
4. Kendall, Sir Maurice and Plackett, R.L., (1977) *Studies In the History of Statistics and Probability.* Vol. 2, pp. 277–333, Macmillan Publishing, New York.
5. Pearson, E.S., *The History of Statistics in the 17th and 18th Centuries.* Macmillan Publishing, New York.
6. Muhlberger, S., (1998) On Line Reference Book for Medieval Studies.
7. Owen, D. B., *On the History of Probability and Statistics.* Marcel Dekker Inc., New York.
8. Bacon, F., (1627) *Sylva sylvarum, or a Natural History.* William Rawley, London.
9. Young, A., (1771) *A Course of Experimental Agriculture.* J. Exshaw et al., Dublin.
10. "Student" 1908 "The Probable Error of a Mean," *Biometrika* 6:1–24.
11. Brownlee, K.A., (1965) *Statistical Theory and Methodology in Science and Engineering,* Second Edition, John Wiley & Sons, New York.
12. Fisher, R. A., *Statistical Methods for Research Workers.* Oliver and Boyd, Edinburg, UK.
13. Fisher, R.A., (1933) "The Arrangement of Field Experiments," *Journal of the Ministry of Agriculture,* September 503–513.
14. Todhunder, L.A., (1949) *History of the Mathematical Theory of Probability.* Else Publishing Company, New York.
15. Birnbaum, A., "On the Foundations of Statistical Inference," *Journal of the American Statistical Association* 57:269–306.
16. Berkson, J., (1942) "Experiences with tests of significance. A reply to R.A. Fisher," *Journal of American Statistical Association* 37:242–246.
17. Berkson, J., (1942) "Test of significance considered as evidence," *Journal of the American Statistical Association* 37:335–345.
18. Fisher, R.A., (1942) "Response to Berkson," *Journal of the American Statistical Association* 37:103–104.
19. Poole, C., (1987) "Beyond the confidence interval," *American Journal of Public Health.* 77:195–199.
20. Poole, C., (1988) "Feelings and Frequencies: Two kinds of probability in public health research," *American Journal of Public Health* 78:1531–1533.
21. Gardner, M.J., and Altman, D.G., (1986) "Confidence intervals rather than p values. Estimation rather than hypothesis testing," *British Medical Journal* 292:746–750.

22. Fleiss, J.L., (1986) "Significance tests have a role in epidemiologic research; reactions to A.M. Walker. (Different Views)," *American Journal of Public Health* 76:559–560.
23. Fleiss, J.L. (1986) "Confidence intervals vs. significance tests: quantitative interpretation. (Letter)," *American Journal of Public Health* 76:587–587.
24. Fleiss, J.L., (1986) "Dr. Fleiss response (Letter)," *American Journal of Public Health* 76:1033–1034.
25. Walker, A.M., (1986) "Reporting the results of epidemiologic studies," *American Journal of Public Health* 76:556–558.
26. Walker, A.M., (1986) "Significance tests [sic] represent consensus and standard practice (Letter)" *American Journal of Public Health* 76:1033–1034. (see also Journal erratum 1986; 76:1087–1088.)
27. Lang, J.M., Rothman, K.L., and Cann, C.L., (1998) "That confounded p value," *Epidemiology* 9:7–8.

1

CHAPTER

Patients, Patience, and *P* Values

This chapter is written for physicians from the perspective of a physician, in recognition that, of all professionals, we as physicians have the greatest philosophical difficulty coming to grips with the concepts of *p* values and sampling error. This is nothing to be ashamed of, however, because we were designed for this confusion.

The Dilemma of Physicians

From our formative medical educational experiences, we physicians are trained to focus our energies on the individual patient to the exclusion of the population. Beginning in medical school, the instruction in anatomy, histology, biochemistry, and physiology we received was not to enhance our understanding of the constitution of the population, but to deepen our understanding of the structure of the individual. We are trained in pharmacology for its application, by and large, to the one patient. We were trained to develop thorough, exhaustive differential diagnoses, compiling a complete list of possible explanations for the symptoms and signs the individual patient presented, no matter how unlikely that explanation might be. In my medical education, a seemingly disproportionate emphasis was placed on the rare diseases of microbiology and pathology (e.g., Whipple's disease or Tsushugamuchi

20

fever), so that my classmates and I could identify the one rare patient who might have the unusual disease. We were taught these uncommon diseases "to bring the rare to bear" as we concentrated on the one patient, not the population. We remember the first patient for whom we ever had the responsibility of performing a history and physical diagnosis. (For me, it was an adult, deaf-mute male at North Shore Hospital on Long Island, New York, in March, 1976.)

Occasionally we were confronted by another perspective, such as a short course in epidemiology or biostatistics in medical school. Although, this short exposure struggled to dig through the single patient perspective, many of us believed with some self-satisfaction that the way to improve a population was by individual physicians treating individual patients one at a time. The global population perspective remained "outside" and foreign to us. We were trained to place the patient in a position of preeminence. We took a patient-oriented oath that insisted on it.

As house officers, we focused not on populations of patients, but on the few (although at the time it seemed like the many) patients on the wards, floors, and units we covered. We attended lectures, asking How will this affect the patients under my care? We built our practices one patient at a time, one family at a time. This is based on the foundation that the most important patient we will see is the one we are treating now. All of our skills and energy must be focused there. The patient places a tremendous burden on us and we are trained and disciplined to bear it. We should not, cannot, dare not turn our faces from this challenge.

Yet it seems that research specialists try to force physicians into embracing concepts we have been specifically trained to shun. The message we hear from many researchers is that the findings in the individual patient are not so important—it is the sample of patients, it is the population of patients, that should dominate. They tell us to focus on the best result for the average patient and not on what's best for an individual. We as physicians know patients are very different from one another, unique in an uncountable number of ways—we try to take advantage of this built-in variability. The research perspective says this variability is a problem to be "adjusted for," "controlled," or even "removed." Perhaps this is not the message researchers mean to transmit, but it all to often the message physicians receive. There has been and will be tension between the individual practice of medicine and the implications of the mathematical tools used to propel medicine forward. We physicians should not turn our faces from this.

Instead, we need to understand this, accept this, and finally to harness it.

Perhaps we can begin by repudiating the idea that individual patient preeminence is negotiable. The patient comes first—the implications of any other policy are both unthinkable and unethical for us and damaging to our patients and their families. However, we must recognize that our focus on the individual patient is exactly what blinds us to an objective view of the effects of our therapies. Thomas Moore [1] has recently reminded us that we as physicians often cannot see the results of our own errors. For example, if patients who respond well to our treatments return to see us, while the poor responders drift away, we are lulled into a false sense of confidence in the utility of the intervention. On the other hand, if patients who improve due to our intervention no longer return to see us, while those who are made worse return to complain and seek additional solutions, we may prematurely abandon an important and promising therapy. Some patients improve (or deteriorate) regardless of what we do. The individual focus that is required of us and that we embrace is what blinds our view of the true benefit of therapy. We require evidence-based medicine, but the evidence we collect from our daily practices is subjective and therefore suspect.

If we therefore must admit that we cannot have an objective assessment of our work, how should we then proceed? Perhaps we should start by responding to the patients' trust in us by reducing our own trust in ourselves. Can it be true that we have too much faith in our own ideas? We are enamoured with theories, e.g., the arrhythmia suppression hypothesis, or the immunotherapy hypothesis for cancer. These theories are well researched at the basic level, are replete with detail and hold out tremendous promise for our patients, and we are easily mesmerized by them. However, from all of the discussions, from all of the anecdotes, from all of the articles, and from all of the working groups, the theory begins to take on a life of its own—and herein lies the great trap. Well-developed theories are often both seductive and wrong, and basing patient practice in a false theory, however attractive that theory is, has had and will continue to have devastating effects on patients, their families, and our communities.

Accepting the conclusion before formally testing it is a wonderful thing in religion, but it is anathema to science. Sometimes it is good for us all to be painfully reminded that for hundreds of years physicians allowed infected wounds to fester because an ancient text declared authoritatively and erroneously that purulence was beneficial. We also are reminded that professional, compassionate doctors who placed their patients first as we do, who were true to their oaths we are, often provided this barbaric treatment. By accepting the patient preeminence philosophy we must also accept the blinding effect this philosophy has on our view of what we do. We must therefore recognize that additional tools are required to allow us to see the effect of therapy more objectively. Thus, understanding the role of the population or the sample does not represent a philosophical replacement but a philosophical addition.

The Great Compromise

A researcher studying a particular disease (say, congestive heart failure), if she could, would study every single patient with that disease—everywhere. She would identify the world population with congestive heart failure, contact each member, and then thoroughly study each one, recording the necessary data required to understand them. This, of course, is quite impossible. Even if she could solve the intractable financial and logistical problem, the fact that many patients would refuse to be studied makes this approach untenable if not patently absurd. Therefore researchers compromise—they give up on the notion of studying every member of the population, replacing it with the concept of thoroughly studying only a sample of the entire population. The advantage of this approach is immediate; the researcher now has a group of patients to study completely—the research program is now executable. However, the researcher pays a price for this executability. She must recognize that, just as she selected a sample, other investigators, equally motivated and equally trained, will draw their own samples from the population. Since their samples will contain different patients, with different life experiences, measurements on these patients will be different from measurements taken from the first investigator's sample of patients. The variability of the same measure across different samples, each generated by the same population is what we call sampling error. Populations will generate many different samples. Since the price the investigator pays for taking one sample is the recognition that different samples, generated by different investigators, generate different results, why should one investigator's findings be believed over another?

Random sampling

When an investigator chooses a sample from a population, he has many selection schemes that he they may follow. The investigator could select all males, for example, or restrict selection to only patients between forty and fifty years of age. The selection criteria are arbitrary but the consequences can be profound. In order to choose the best criteria for selecting patients, we must remember that we rely on the sample to contain, reflect, and therefore reveal relationships that exist in the population. The only purpose the sample serves, therefore, is to represent the population. The sample is our view of the population. If that view is blurred, bent, or otherwise distorted, we have difficulty discerning what is going on in the population from what we see in our sample. We must choose our sample in the way that provides the clearest view of the population.

The clearest view of the population is provided if the sample is selected randomly. To most people, the word *random* is associated with chaos. It refers to a thing that is unstructured, unplanned, directionless, and haphazard. Perhaps that is so for many events we deal with in the world, but it is not true for random sampling schemes. Applying simple random selection in choosing a sample simply means that every patient in the population has the same, constant chance of being selected for the sample The simple random sampling plan, by giving each population member the same constant probability of gaining entry to the sample, will many times yield a sample that is representative of the population, and findings generated from the sample will be truly reflective of findings in the population.

Now, what does *reflective* mean? Even a random sample, though it is planned, representative, and laudable, is, after all, just a single sample—it may not contain the truth about a population. Let's examine the effect of sampling error in a population.

Example of sampling error

To understand the different views a sample can provide of a population, let's carry out an artificial experiment. Consider that there is a population of 2231 patients who are at risk for a disease. This collection of 2231 patients represents all of the patients in the world at risk for this disease. The investigators will sample

Table 1.1. Investigator's Results

| | Number of patients | | | |
	Placebo	Active	Total	Relative Risk
Number of Deaths	25	29	54	
Total Patients	109	107	216	
Death Rate	0.229	0.271	0.250	1.21

from this population.[1] The effect of a therapy for the disease in this population is that the risk of death is reduced by 20 percent (i.e. 20 percent of the deaths which would have occurred without therapy are now prevented). This is the "true state of nature". The investigator deems to know this but cannot since he only samples a fraction of these patients.

Now consider an investigator who does not know the true state of nature. The best that he can do is to take a random sample from this population and study the effect of the therapy. The investigator draws a sample of 216 patients from this population of 2231, and observes the results (Table 1.1).

In this one sample, there were 25 deaths in the placebo group and 29 deaths in the active group, an excess of four deaths attributable to active therapy. The cumulative mortality rate for the placebo group is 0.229 (25/109) for the placebo group and 0.271 (29/107) for the active group. The relative risk of therapy[2] is 1.21. If the therapy were neutral, causing no more deaths in the active group than in the placebo group, the relative risk would be 1.00. The value of 1.21 suggests that therapy may be harmful, causing 21 percent more deaths in the treatment group than in the placebo group.

The promulgation of these results in the medical literature, at symposiums, at workshops, and conferences would suggest that the therapy is not helpful, and in fact is harmful. Many cardiologists would labor to explain these surprising findings (possible explanations would be that the study explicitly excluded patients who would be helped by the study, or that the cause specific death rates should be examined to see if patients died of events

---

[1] We rarely have an opportunity to view an entire population, but we will take a liberty here for illustrative purposes.

[2] The relative risk is computed using Cox proportional hazard regression analysis, a computational detail that is not necessary for the comprehension of this discussion.

not influenced by the therapy). Some would theorize that perhaps the therapy itself did beneficially affect the course of the disease, but produced another unanticipated harmful effect that was fatal. Experienced academicians and researchers have watched this scenario play out in many circumstances. However, the role of sampling error is insidious. Let's see the results of other samples taken from this same population of 2231 patients.

The sampling variability is stunning (Table 1.2). In the population of 2231 in which the therapy is in fact known to be effective, five of the ten small samples suggest a harmful effect. On the other hand, Sample 3 suggests a powerful beneficial therapy effect (relative risk in sample three is 0.52, suggesting a $1 - 0.52 = 48$ percent reduction in death afforded by the therapy). Sample 5 suggests a 43 percent increase in deaths. Imagine if these ten samples reflected the results of each of ten investigators, one investigator to a sample. These investigators at a meeting would provide often long and sometimes loud commentary as they labored to justify their own findings, each investigator broadcasting his own findings and coming up with criticisms of the other investigators' conclusions. The "random" in random sampling may not be chaotic, but this resulting situation surely is, and the confusion is solely due to sampling error.

This example demonstrates that, even with a random sample, it is possible that one clear relationship in the population will not be mirrored in the sampling results. In fact, we would have trouble identifying the true relationship between therapy and total mortality by looking at the ten sample results. This is why sampling variability is so dangerous to investigators. A clinician copes with the variability of a patient's response to a drug by using the traditional tools of clinical practice available to her. These tools include taking a family history, examining the patient's previous exposure to this class of drugs, and remaining vigilant in watching for the occurrence of any adverse reaction. We need new tools to help us with sampling error so that we can assess the impact of the therapy in the community.

Fleas

Sampling error is the bane of the researcher's efforts. Research efforts that can include and study every single member of the pop-

Table 1.2. Results of Ten Samples Drawn at Random from a
Population with a relative risk of therapy = 0.81

		Number of Patients			Relative
	Variable	Placebo	Active	Total	Risk
Sample 1	Number of Deaths	25	29	54	
	Total Patients	109	107	216	
	Death Rate	0.229	0.271	0.25	1.21
Sample 2	Total Mortality	24	22	46	
	At Risk	115	99	214	
	Cum Inc Rate	0.209	0.222	0.215	1.13
Sample 3	Total Mortality	35	15	50	
	At Risk	122	92	214	
	Cum Inc Rate	0.287	0.163	0.234	0.52
Sample 4	Total Mortality	25	30	55	
	At Risk	107	95	202	
	Cum Inc Rate	0.234	0.316	0.272	1.43
Sample 5	Total Mortality	31	17	48	
	At Risk	112	96	208	
	Cum Inc Rate	0.277	0.177	0.231	0.62
Sample 6	Total Mortality	26	27	53	
	At Risk	103	110	213	
	Cum Inc Rate	0.252	0.245	0.249	1.02
Sample 7	Total Mortality	27	24	51	
	At Risk	104	106	210	
	Cum Inc Rate	0.26	0.226	0.243	0.88
Sample 8	Total Mortality	24	20	44	
	At Risk	92	92	184	
	Cum Inc Rate	0.261	0.217	0.239	0.82
Sample 9	Total Mortality	31	20	51	
	At Risk	110	99	209	
	Cum Inc Rate	0.282	0.202	0.244	0.69
Sample 10	Total Mortality	24	26	50	
	At Risk	98	91	189	
	Cum Inc Rate	0.245	0.286	0.265	1.01

ulation of interest are more easily designed, more easily executed, more easily analyzed, and certainly more easily interpreted. However, what makes our sampling based studies executable (i.e. the sampling plan) is precisely what introduces sampling error and its implications into our effort. Consider the following passage from the novel *Arrowsmith* by Sinclair Lewis (page 365).[3] The quote is from Sondelius, an epidemiologist, dying from bubonic plague, for which the flea is a vector in the disease transmission.

> Gottlieb is right about these jests of God. Yeh! His best one is the tropics. God planned them so beautiful, flowers and sea and mountains. He made the fruit to grow so well that man need not work—and then He laughed, and stuck in volcanoes and snakes and damp heat and early senility and the plague and malaria. But the nastiest trick He ever played on man was inventing the flea.

Sampling error is the flea of our research tropics. We can't get rid of it, but we enjoy the tropics too much to leave.

Being Dealt a Bad Hand

Remember that in the previous example, we know the true state of nature for the therapy—total mortality relationship in the population. Why was this notion of a therapy benefit not successfully transmitted to each of the random samples? Under random sampling schemes, many of the samples will be representative of the population. However, despite the investigator's best efforts, the population will sometimes "deal him a bad hand," i.e. provide a sample whose findings of efficacy will not reflect the findings in the population at large. Sometimes, just through the play of chance, the sample will contain data (in Sample 4 above) suggesting a harmful effect of therapy. The problem is, in one experiment we have only one sample. Given this established level of variability, how do we decide whether the sample is true to the findings in the population or just the result of a "bad hand"? The *p* value answers this question. It gives us the probability that we do not have a representative sample. The *p* value (also known as

---

[3] A fine novel about the development of a medical researcher [2].

alpha error or the probability of type I error) is the probability that a population in which there is no relationship between the treatment and the disease produces a sample that suggests such a relationship exists. This sample based evidence of a relationship is present just through the play of chance. The population misled us by producing an unrepresentative picture of itself. The p value is the probability we have been misled in this fashion. That's all it is.

There is a difference between p values and alpha levels. Alpha levels are prospectively allocated before the study begins. P values are measured experimentally at the end of the study, and compared to the alpha level that was set at the study's inception.

Therefore, if we have a sample which suggests a relationship exists between treatment and disease, the smaller the p value in that sample, the more confident we can be that we have not been misled by the population—the more confident we can be that our sample is representative of the population, and that the relationship between treatment and disease truly exists in the population.

Let's examine this further. For the above experiment, we know the therapy produces a 20 percent reduction in total mortality for the population. Returning to investigator 1, we see a 21 percent increase in total mortality associated with the therapy. Now the population has done one of two things for investigator 1. Either there is a 21 percent increase in total mortality in the population (we know this is not the case, but the investigator only knows his sample) and Investigator 1's sample accurately reflects the population, or the population does not have a 21 percent increase in total mortality, but has fooled Investigator 1 by providing a misleading and unrepresentative sample. The p value is the probability that the population generated an unrepresentative sample. In this case the p value is 0.250. This means that if there is no harmful effect of the drug in the population, then there is one chance in four that the population has dealt him a bad hand, producing this finding of 21 percent harm. Since we would be fooled one time in four if we believe the result of the sample, we disregard the sample result. Let's return to examine the ten investigators' findings, now including the p values (Table 1.3).

The p values shed additional light on the findings of the investigators. For nine out of ten of them, to believe their results, we must accept a high probability of being misled by the population. The only sample that has a relatively small p value and a high likelihood of truly reflecting the therapy—total mortality relationship in the sample is sample 3, suggesting a benefit.

Table 1.3. Results of Ten Samples Drawn at Random from a Population with a Relative Risk of Therapy = 0.81

| | Number of Patients | | | | |
Variable	Placebo	Active	Total	P Value	Relative Risk
Sample 1					
Number of Deaths	25	29	54		
Total Patients	109	107	216		
Death Rate	0.229	0.271	0.25	0.476	1.21
Sample 2					
Total Mortality	24	22	46		
At Risk	115	99	214		
Cum Inc Rate	0.209	0.222	0.215	0.676	1.13
Sample 3					
Total Mortality	35	15	50		
At Risk	122	92	214		
Cum Inc Rate	0.287	0.163	0.234	0.033	0.52
Sample 4					
Total Mortality	25	30	55		
At Risk	107	95	202		
Cum Inc Rate	0.234	0.316	0.272	0.186	1.43
Sample 5					
Total Mortality	31	17	48		
At Risk	112	96	208		
Cum Inc Rate	0.277	0.177	0.231	0.108	0.62
Sample 6					
Total Mortality	26	27	53		
At Risk	103	110	213		
Cum Inc Rate	0.252	0.245	0.249	0.942	1.02

Table 1.3. (Continued).

		Number of Patients				
	Variable	Placebo	Active	Total	P Value	Relative Risk
Sample 7	Total Mortality	27	24	51		
	At Risk	104	106	210		
	Cum Inc Rate	0.26	0.226	0.243	0.650	0.88
Sample 8	Total Mortality	24	20	44		
	At Risk	92	92	184		
	Cum Inc Rate	0.261	0.217	0.239	0.507	0.82
Sample 9	Total Mortality	31	20	51		
	At Risk	110	99	209		
	Cum Inc Rate	0.282	0.202	0.244	0.201	0.69
Sample 10	Total Mortality	24	26	50		
	At Risk	98	91	189		
	Cum Inc Rate	0.245	0.286	0.265	0.536	1.01

So we have seen that sampling error is dangerous to the integrity of the experiment and, if handled inappropriately, critically weakens the investigators' abilities to generalize their findings to the larger population from which the sample was drawn. However, by the very nature of a sample, the researcher must cope with sampling error. The *p* value handles this sampling error by linking the experiment's outcome to the types of samples the population may have produced. We may think of the *p* value as the repository of sampling error in the experiment. We try to reduce sampling error as best we can, but in the end we have to incorporate it into our conclusions. The *p* value is this incorporation. The p value provides an important link between the results in the sample and the "true state of nature" in the population from which the sample was derived.[4]

Leaky Protocols and Sampling Error Contamination

If executed correctly, a research program will obtain its sample of data randomly, channeling this sampling error to the type I and type II errors. However, there are other destinations this sampling error could find, with devastating implications for the interpretation of the experiment. Consider the following hypothetical example.

An enthusiastic young researcher, Catalina, is interested in demonstrating the progressive deterioration in heart function observed in patients with mild congestive heart failure. She has designed a research program to examine the change in left ventricular ejection volume over time. Catalina recruits her sample randomly over two years from the population of people with congestive heart failure, and follows each patient for five years, measuring heart function at baseline (i.e., when the patient agrees to enter the study) and five years later. Although Catalina is focused

---

[4] If the experiment produces a large *p* value, the investigator must now be concerned about the possibility that the population does demonstrate an effect of therapy, but has misled the investigators by dealing them an unrepresentative sample. This is called a beta error or Type II error discussed in chapter five. The important point here is that both alpha and beta errors are designed to measure the effect of sampling error—nothing more.

on the change in left ventricular ejection fraction (LVEF), she also collects other measures of left ventricular dysfunction. These include end diastolic volume, end systolic volume, stroke volume, and cardiac output.

At the study's conclusion, Catalina examines her data with great anticipation. She compares the baseline findings to the five-year findings for all of the patients and, to her surprise and horror, discovers that there has not been an important change in LVEF. This is quite a shock to her, since she expected a substantial decrease in LVEF over the five years of follow-up. She also notices, however, that although the LVEF measurements have not decreased end diastolic volumes (EDV) have changed substantially. She therefore decides to change the endpoint for the program from LVEF to EDV and to characterize the deterioration of her patients in terms of EDV, thoroughly analyzing it, saying nothing in the end about ejection fraction.

Some researchers would have no problem with Catalina's last minute endpoint change. They would argue that end diastolic volume and left ventricular ejection reflect measurements of the same underlying pathophysiology; since they jointly measure the progress of the same disease process, they should be interchangeable as endpoints. Others would see that this endpoint change is wrong, but may be unclear as to exactly what the problem is. They would say that the decision to change the endpoint was "data driven." Well, what's so wrong with that? Aren't the results of any study "data driven"? What's wrong is that the random data have been permitted to convert the fixed research plan of evaluating LVEF to a random plan, (i.e., random data produced a fortuitous change in EDV, so now analyse this randomly chosen endpoint that was selected by the data). The study, which first contained a fixed analysis plan of random data, is now a random analysis of random data.

The decision to change the endpoint from LVEF to EDV was based solely on the findings in the sample. Why didn't LVEF change as Catalina anticipated? While it is true that one explanation would be that, in the population, the LVEF doesn't change over time, another explanation is that LVEF does decrease in the population, but that the population produced an unrepresentative sample for her. But, with the endpoint change from LVEF to EDV, our ability to capture and identify sampling error is destroyed. Let's say that another investigator (Susi) sampled from the same population as Catalina, but in the examination of her sample,

neither LVEF nor EDV showed evidence of change but end systolic volume (ESV) did. Susi then changes her endpoint from
LVEF to (ESV), rejecting LVEF. Let's also consider that Al, a third
investigator, again sampling from the same population, notices,
that it is stroke volume (SV), not left ventricular ejection fraction,
nor EDV, nor ESV that shows promise of change. Al chooses to
report the findings of the trial for stroke volume. Three different
researchers report three different findings, (Catalina reports EDV,
Susi reports ESV, and Al reports SV). Nobody reports LVEF, which
was the prospectively identified endpoint chosen by each of these
researchers.

How can these results be interpreted? In each of these three
research programs, there are now two sources of variability
where there was only supposed to be one. The first source of
variability is the variability of the measurements from subject to
subject—this was easily anticipated. Computing the standard deviation of the measurement and constructing a test statistic, converting it to a _p_ value, appropriately incorporates this subject-to-
subject variability. However, there is another source of variation
that was never anticipated–the variability in endpoint selection.
Each investigator chose a different endpoint based on their individual dataset—however, each of these datasets contained sampling variability that is random. Since sampling variability led to
the prominence and selection of the each of their new endpoints,
the endpoint selection procedure was a random process. We
know how to compute the variability of a measurement changes
from subject to subject, but how do we go about computing the
variability of the endpoint selection process? We can't—we have
no good way to do this. The _p_ value should be simply a measure
of sampling error. However, because of the changes in endpoints,
the _p_ value has bound up in it both sampling error and the variability of the endpoint selection process. It was not constructed to
handle both, and so cannot be interpreted. Here the non-sampling
variability (i.e., variability in endpoint) destroyed the experiment's interpretation.

There are two maneuvers investigators can appropriately execute to control sampling error. The first tack that they can take is
to reduce it by making precise measurement estimates. They use
well-renowned labs for serum measurements. They measure
clinical parameters by relying on skilled professionals who have
undergone standardized training. They use an endpoint committee for endpoint determinations. All these approaches are impor-

tant and valuable because they reduce intersubject variability. The second maneuver is to channel the sampling error through a tight protocol that resists changes due to sampling error, protecting the execution and analysis procedures from the ravages of random variability. The repositories for this sampling error are the type I and type II errors. The previous, hypothetical study of Catalina et al. was designed with one source of variability (the intersubject differences in the endpoint measurement), but now has a new source of variability—that of endpoint choice. This variability is random as well. The first source of randomization can be reduced and channeled. The second source cannot be channeled and, since it was not reduced, it rises up to strangle the research program's interpretation. The only way to effectively deal with this source of variability is to control it—make a prospective (i.e., before the study begins, during the planning stage) choice for the endpoint, allowing no variability at all. In this case, that means to choose one endpoint measure and stick with it.

Frankly, this rigidity about protocol changes frankly sticks in the throats of many physician investigators. After all, don't we as physician-investigators have the right to change the endpoint when confronted by surprising information? In fact, some of us feel that this flexibility, this adaptability to rapidly shift the direction of the study based on the data is a useful skill. Unfortunately, these swift, agile responses to changing data patterns are most often chasing only the patternless, random sample variability and will, after great effort, produce a product of little of value. Like a high performance sports car driving furiously around and around in a circular driveway, lots of energy produces little real constructive movement.

Trying to "adjust" an experiment in the middle of execution is often hazardous, causing much unintentional harm. Consider the following.

A thirty-four-year-old automobile mechanic from Alamo, Michigan was troubled by a noise coming from the truck he and his friend were driving. The mechanic insisted on finding the noise's source. Instructing his friend to continue driving so the noise would continue, the mechanic maneuvered outside of the truck and then—while the truck was still being driven—continued to squirm and maneuver until he was underneath the truck. While carrying out his investigation, his clothing caught on part of the undercarriage. Some miles later when his friend finally stopped the car and got out, he found the mechanic "wrapped in the drive shaft"—quite dead.

When tempted to change a research program once underway, don't get wrapped in the drive shaft.

Study Concordance vs. Study Discordance

As we have seen, the *p* value of an experiment is relevant to the scientific community if the *p* value is the only repository of that experiment's sampling error, i.e., it is the result of a well-defined, prospectively fixed experiment whose only random component is the data itself. This is not the case when the investigators allow sampling error to affect the conduct of an experiment, as in the example above. If the data generated by the experiment are allowed to influence the experiment (e.g., lead the investigators to change the experiment's endpoint), then the experiment has an unanticipated random component. Since the random data have been allowed to transmit randomness to the analysis plan and the research program's results, the *p* value is meaningless since it is the result not just of random data, but of a random analysis plan.

The *p* value is useful to us only if it represents a population-based sampling event of interest to the scientific community and the experiment is carried out per protocol independent of the data collected. Define study concordance [3] as the execution of a research effort in accordance with a prespecified protocol. With study concordance, the type I error contains all of the sampling error, and the *p* value of the experiment answers the question raised by the research community. When the data are allowed to alter the experiment's execution, and discrepancies are created between the protocol's plan of operation and the research program's actual execution occur, study discordance exists, and the sampling error has influenced not just the data, but the analysis plan.

The notion of study discordance is not "all or none." Every study encounters an unanticipated occurrence, and some discordance is present in every research program. However, if the discordance is mild, most of the sampling error is contained in the *p* value and only a minor adjustment is required. However, if there is severe or profound study discordance, the study's p value may be of little value. Severe study discordance can unfortunately be lethal to the interpretation of a research program's results, since it produces a random experiment with an uninterpretable, corrupt p value.[5] It is not our goal here to discuss how to adjust the p value. Our goal is to recognize study discordance and classify it as mild or severe.

Mild Experimental Discordance — Study P Value Adjustment

Most research programs contain some study discordance. In these circumstances, the study p value can be adjusted easily. Consider the protocol for a prospectively designed, double-blind, randomized, controlled clinical trial to assess an intervention for improving survival in patients with myocardial infarction. The experiment's planners determine that a sample size of 2,182 patients is required.[6] However, suppose only 2,000 patients are randomized, representing a discrepancy with the experimental plan. At the study's conclusion, the p value is 0.01. Is the experiment destroyed by the smaller-than-anticipated sample size? Our intuition tells us this experiment (if positive) is still interpretable. The discrepancy is relatively minor (a reduction in sample size from 2,182 to 2,000). How much less clear is our view of the treatment effect in the population from a sample of 2,000 than from a slightly larger sample of 2,182? Or, as the investigators' critics would ask, "Are these investigators much more likely to be misled by a sample size of 2,000 then by a sample size of 2,182?" The answer is, perhaps a little bit more, but not much. Since the computation for the p value includes sample size, the new sample size would be incorporated into the value computation. Note that the formula for the analysis and the p value computations have not changed. The analysis plan remains fixed. The view of the population from the sample is relatively uncluttered and the p value's interpretation remains clear.

Mild Discordance in Subgroup Size

Consider a research program designed to assess the impact of various non-pharmacologic and pharmacologic measures to control blood pressure. In order to have the widest possible general-

---

[5] In a negative study, in which attention often focuses on power, the beta error is corrupted as a result of experimental discordance.

[6] How to construct the sample size is discussed in chapter 5.

izability of these findings, the investigators state in the protocol their prospective plan to select a simple random sample, 60 percent of which will consist of patients of African-American descent. The investigators realize that the size of the African-American subcohort will not allow them to draw as clear a set of conclusions as they will from the larger main study, but they desire to have a credible argument for extending the findings of the trial to the African-American population. However, during the execution of the trial, despite the investigators' best efforts, African-American recruitment falls short of expectations, and the proportion of the sample that is African-American is only 0.40. Although many readers would decry the shortfall, in general there would be no objections to extending the findings of the experiment to African-American patients. There was no change in the procedure to be followed to analyze these patients. The population generated fewer African American patients than anticipated, but the protocol remained fixed and the analysis plan was unchanged. We are slightly more likely to have a skewed view of the African-American population from a sample that is 40 percent African American than from one which is 60 percent African-American[7]. However, if the investigators responded to this lower proportion of African American patients by changing the protocol to improve patient recruitment, e.g., by relaxing entry criteria, or accepting low quality recruiting centers that had first been rejected, the experiment's concordance has decreased to the level of p value corruption.

Severe Discordance

Severe study discordance describes the situation where the research execution has been so different from that prescribed in the prospectively written protocol that the sample provides a hopelessly blurred and distorted view of the population from which it was chosen. P values from these discordant studies are rendered meaningless and irrelevant to the medical community, since the view of the population through the sample is smeared and distorted. This unfortunate state of affairs can be produced by the flawed execution of a well-written protocol. The situation can be so complicated that, in the case of a positive study, the value cannot be computed without controversy. We use the term alpha corruption to signify that the protocol specified alpha error cannot

---

[7] In a negative study, where the issue of power is the critical consideration, beta corruption is the relevant term. See chapter 5 for a discussion of power.

be approximated by the study p value.[8] Experiments that lead to sampling error corruption are essentially useless to the research community.

Consider the case of a clinical trial with two treatment arms designed to assign therapy or placebo randomly and follow patients for four years, hoping to detect a significant benefit for total mortality. However, at the conclusion of the study, 25 percent of patients are lost to follow-up. The implications of this discordance are substantial, because the follow-up losses blur our view of the population. How should the analysis be carried out? The problem here is not that the p value is data based (every p value is data based). The problem introduced by severe study discordance is that the *method* of computing the p value is data based. Should the computation assume that all patients lost to follow-up are dead? Should it assume that patients who are lost to follow-up in the active group are dead, and those who were lost to follow-up and in the placebo group are alive? Should it assume that an equal fraction of patients who are lost to follow-up are alive, regardless of the therapy group assignment? The best choice from among these possibilities is not dictated by the protocol. Instead, the choice of computation is based on belief and the data, itself full of sampling error. Variability has wrenched control of the p value computational procedure from the protocol and dooms this study's interpretation.

The degree of discordance here depends on the magnitude of the p value. If the p value remained below the threshold of significance when we assume all lost patients assigned to the placebo group were alive and all lost patients in the active group were dead, we must conclude the discordance is mild because the worst implications of the follow-up losses do not vitiate the results and the type I error event is still relevant to the scientific community. However, if the p value fluctuates wildly, we may say the discordance is severe and the alpha error corrupted.

Another example of severe study discordance would be the following clinical trial designed to assess the effect of an intervention on patients who have established heart failure at the time of randomization. Patients are randomized to each of a placebo or an active intervention. The prospectively specified endpoint is a

---

[8] We signify alpha error as the type I error allocated to the hypothesis test *a priori* and the p value is actual type I error based on the test statistic constructed at the experiment's conclusion

change in background medication for heart failure (e.g., increase in diuretic use during the trial, or the addition of anticonverting enzyme inhibitor therapy during the trial), a change that would be triggered by deterioration of the patient's left ventricular function over time. The trial requires a sample of 482 patients to be reasonably assured of identifying a 30 percent reduction from a 40 percent cumulative incidence rate of heart failure progression in the population with 80 percent power for a two-sided alpha error rate of 0.05. If the experiment is positive, critics would know that there is only a 5 percent chance that a population of patients with heart failure who would show a 30 percent benefit from this therapy would produce a sample which showed no benefit.

The trial protocol assumes that all patients will have an endpoint assessment. However, during the trial's execution, 60 percent of the patients have missing medical records precluding the determination of endpoint status for them, and allowing endpoint computation on only the remaining 40 percent. Is this experiment interpretable? Can we carry out any posttrial maneuver to make this experiment once again meaningful to the medical community? The waiting scientific world wanted the assurance that the sample would provide a clear view of the population. Clearly, that view is distorted if 60 percent of the sample has missing endpoint information. As before, there is disagreement on the computation of the trial's *p* value, since different assumptions about the medication records for the 60 percent of patients with missing endpoint information would lead to different *p* value computation (Should the *p* value be computed assuming these patients had no endpoints? Assuming only active patients had endpoints?) Each assumption leads to a different *p* value. Experimental discordance is extreme, and the *p* value corruption has profoundly distorted any clear interpretation of the study.

As a final example of discordance, consider the findings of the National Surgical Adjuvant Breast Project (NSABP) [3–4]. This study examined the effect of different therapies for breast cancer reduction. After the study's results were analyzed and published, it was discovered that 99 ineligible patients were deliberately randomized with falsified data. Is this experiment hopelessly corrupted? Should the *p* value formula now change, excluding these patients? One way to resolve this would be to examine whether the *p* value changes much by excluding these ninety nine patients. To assess the experimental discordance produced by this event, one might first examine the trial results excluding these 99 patients. If their exclusion moved the *p* value across the significance threshold, the inclusion of these patients produces unacceptable discordance. However, a second relevant question of the interpretation of the trial must be addressed since the presence of fraudulent data admits the possibility of dishonest behavior elsewhere in the trial apparatus. To address this issue, a full audit of the study data was carried out by Christian et al [5] that could be viewed as an investigation into the degree of discordance. Since the protocol discrepancies identified were small in number and magnitude, the degree of discordance was mild.

Importance of prospective experimental design

Clear *p* value interpretation requires *both* a random sampling plan and a non random study execution and analysis (study concordance). Successful experiments protect study concordance. This concordance is easily lost if data collected during the study are allowed to affect analytical decisions in an unplanned manner, thus allowing sampling error to besmirch protocol-mandated procedures. Since sampling error is a necessary evil in clinical trials, it must be handled with care, insuring that it does not contaminate the research program. Sampling error containment is assured by preventing trial execution decisions from being affected by the data of the experiment. This allows the sampling error to pass through the experiment, being measured in the end by type I and type II errors (Figure 1.1).

The one acceptable repository for sampling error is the type I and type II event probabilities, since they are constructed as sampling error probabilities.

Physician-scientist Community Responsibility

Why should physicians who have been trained to be patient-focused now have to deal with *p* values? Why should alpha

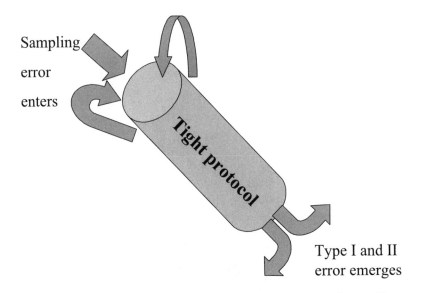

Figure 1.1. Conversion of sampling error to type I and type II error throught tight protocol

considerations be added to our burdens? As stated early in this chapter, this new concern should not replace our patient-oriented philosophy but should augment it. Begin by recognizing that physician scientists bear two preeminent responsibilities. Our first is, of course, to provide the best care for the patients in their research investigations. This is consistent with our oath and is expected. However, since this patient perspective blinds physicians to the effect of their therapies, investigators also have an obligation to protect the populations to which they hope to generalize their results. Promulgating false positive results to the community at large can be calamitous, since it all too easily results in subjecting patients to medications offering no benefit but inflicting significant side effects, inappropriately affecting the community pattern of care.

A prime example of the harm that comes from inadequate population protection is one of the results from the Multiple Risk Factor Intervention Trial (MRFIT)[6] study. Published in 1982, it was a study intended to demonstrate that reductions in the risk factors associated with atherosclerotic cardiovascular disease would be translated into reduction in clinical events, e.g., myocardial infarction and stroke. Patients in the intervention group received treatment for elevated blood pressure, joined cigarette smoking cessation programs, reduced their weight, and lowered their serum lipid levels. At the conclusion of the study, the investigators found and reported that there was no difference in clinical outcome between those patients who received risk factor intervention and those who did not.

These negative findings were a disappointment to the risk factor interventionists, who then poured over the data to identify if any effect could be found in a fraction of the patients randomized. They found one, and it was a bombshell. When the researches ignored the results in the entire randomized cohort (i.e., all randomized patients), and concentrated on those men who were hypertensive, and had resting electrocardiograph (ECG) abnormalities at baseline, they discovered that these patients had a worse outcome when randomized to anti-hypertensive therapy than those who received no such therapy.

Imagine the impact of these findings. At this time in clinical medicine, the importance of identification and treatment of hypertension galvanized physicians. They received instruction on the administration of therapy, new drugs e.g., alphamethyldopa, and clonidine, for the hypertensive patient became available. All of the necessary forces for a war on undiagnosed and untreated hypertension were maneuvering into position when the MRFIT analyses were released. This finding slowed the momentum for the treatment of hypertension. Maybe not all hypertension was bad after all? Maybe hypertensive disease itself was bad, but the treatment was worse?

The real question to be addressed was "Is it just a sampling error?" For years after this finding, clinical trials in hypertension were forced to address this unusual finding. None of the major ones ever reproduced this finding that hypertensive men with resting ECG abnormalities were better off when their hypertension remained unchecked[9]. Nevertheless, a sampling error produced substantial interruption in the treatment of a deadly cardiovascular disease. The community suffered because of inadequate alpha error protection.

Early in this chapter the tools an individual physician uses to protect his patients were mentioned (family history, vigilance in watching for side effects). Health care workers and researchers must understand the utility of type I and type II errors when measured in concordant studies as population protection tools

[9] The admonition of the eighteenth century agriculturist James Johnson are relevant here- see the Prologue.

and require that these tools be wielded appropriately by physician investigators. Only if these are produced from (1) methodologically concordant experiment utilizing a random sample and, (2) occur at a tolerably low rate can the community be assured that the conclusions of the trial most likely reflect the anticipated experience of the patient community.

Patience and Tight Protocols

The development of a tight protocol, immune to unplanned sampling error contamination, is a praiseworthy effort but takes a substantial amount of time and requires great patience. The investigators who are designing the study must have the patience to design the trial appropriately. They must take the time to understand the population from which they will sample. They must take the time to make a focused determination of the necessary endpoint measurements. They must take the time to assess endpoint measures accurately and precisely. Sometimes, they must have the patience to carry out a small pilot study, postponing the main trial until they have tested recruitment and data collection strategies. Those who make these efforts are rewarded with well considered protocols that are executable, and have a clearly articulated analysis plan that is data independent. Investigators may profit from remembering the Quaker admonition "strength in this life, happiness in the next."

After the protocol is written and accepted, investigators must insist on nothing less than its rigorous execution. The protocol is the rule book of the trial, and all involved must strictly adhere to it. Information about a violation of the trial protocol must immediately raise concerns for the presence of study discordance with attendant alpha error corruption.

Discovering a New World

This notion of "First say what you'll do, then do what you said" is unfortunately undigestable to many in health care. They believe this policy disparages the importance of serendipitous discovery, and react strongly against any principle which may tend to belittle this important scientific tool of discovery. This was forcefully announced at a meeting with representatives of a drug company during which I ennunciated the importance of prospective statements in experimental design. One drug company executive stood up and challenged me, stating that he could never accept this principle. Why, he pointed out, if Columbus had followed this preannouncement rule, he could never claim that he discovered the new world, since he found it by accident![10].

The supremacy of a hypothesis driven research does not denigrate surprizes. Quite the contrary, we learn by surprizes in science. The key features of our principle are (1) we cannot blindly take every finding in a sample and extend that finding to a much larger population and (2) the magnitude of the p value by itself does not determine which finding should be extended to the population, and which should be left behind in the sample. The findings for which the experiment was designed are most likely to be the generalizable findings—it is those we take to the population with us. The research design is not random; it is rigidly laid to answer certain questions, and it is those answers (be they good or bad) that should play the predominant role in reporting the medical research. Other findings in the sample should not be ignored just because they were prospectively identified. They should be reported, but as the result of exploratory analyses. Thus, in reporting findings from experiments, it is best to first report the findings of those which were the basis of prospective statements, on which some prior type I error has been allocated. Once this has been completed, the researcher may announce other unexpected findings, but with the preample that these are exploratory findings. These exploratory findings are disseminated to raise new questions not to answer them. To enforce this point, these exploratory, or hypothesis generating results should be reported without p-values. Z scores[11] would suffice very nicely here, since they provide a normed effect size, without mixing in the sampling error issue which is diffcult to interpret in the absence of a prospective statement and prior alpha allocation.

---

[10] This is a very amusing example of a serious issue. Clearly, Columbus was not taking a sample. Even so, his "hypothesis generating" discovery had to be confirmed with successive trips, both by himself (he made three additional voyages) and by others before the concept of a New World was established.

[11] If the probability distribution of the test statistic does not follow a standard normal distribution, the test statistic itself could be reported.

Conclusions

Sampling error is a necessary evil in research programs. Left unchecked, unreduced and unchanneled, it will wreck the research plan, making the study's conclusions uninterpretable. Vigilant investigators must remain on the lookout for sampling error's ability to corrupt the experiment. Discordant program execution will open the study to the corrosive effects of sampling error, turning the program into an uninterpretable, unusable husk. As we interpret research program *p* values, we should be on the alert for changes in trial execution. Such data driven protocol deviations, are a klaxon for alpha and beta error contamination. Slurring the interpretation of *p* values through study discordance makes the view of the population through the sample unusable and the study a failure. Investigators should simply plan what they wish to do, then do precisely what they planned.

Finally, community protection is paramount. Even with adequate precaution sampling error can still result in the wrong conclusion. Physicians must be ever suspicious of what we think we know and must ride herd over our inclination to explain any research result. Ask first if these results are due to sampling error. If they are, we need not go forward with interesting theories for the research findings, since that would be trying to explain random data patterns, and our time could be better used elsewhere.

References

1. Moore, T., (1995) *Deadly Medicine*. Simon and Schuster, New York.
2. Lewis, S., (1953) *Arrowsmith*. Brace and World Inc, Harcourt.
3. Moye, L.A., (1998) "P value interpretation and alpha allocation in clinical trials," *Annals of Epidemiology* 8:351–357.
4. Fisher, B., Bauer, M., and Margolese R., (1985) "Eight year results of a randomized clinical trial comparing total mastectomy and segmental mastectomy with or without radiation in the treatment of breast cancer," *N Engl J Med* 312:665–673.
5. Fisher, B., Bauer, M., and Margolese R., (1985) "Eight year results of a randomized clinical trial comparing total mastectomy and segmental mastectomy with or without radiation in the treatment of breast cancer," *N Engl J Med* 320:822–828.

6. Christian, M.C., Mccabe M.S., Korn, E.L., Abrams J.S., Kaplan, R.S., and Friedman, M.A., (1995), "The National Cancer Institute audit of the national surgical adjuvant breast and bowel project protocol B-06," *N Engl J Med* 333:1469–1474.

7. MRFIT Investigators. (1982) "Multiple risk factor intervention trial," *Journal of the American Medical Association* 248:1465–1477.

2

Shrine Worship

The Common Nightmare

Here is one variation on a common nightmare of all investigators.

After years of practice and careful observation, a distinguished physician developed a theory for the treatment of a disease. A time of arduous work followed, during which he convinced his colleagues of the truth of his thesis, worked patiently to build a funding base, and assembled a cadre of investigators. Finally, he was in a position to put his clinical hypothesis to the definitive test through a formal, randomized, double-blind, placebo-controlled clinical trial. Several more years of diligent and patient work elapsed as the trial was executed, during which time our scientist could only watch from the sidelines. Finally, after many seasons, the trial concluded and its results were revealed. The therapy produced the desired beneficial effect, however, the p value was 0.06. As the implications of this insignificant finding broke through to the investigator, he, in absolute frustration and despair exclaimed "why must we worship at the shrine of 0.05?"[1]

By the end of this chapter we will have provided some sound advice to this investigator without resorting to what is often seen as statistical doubletalk. But first, let's feel his pain.

[1] Taken from a story related by Eugene Braunwald.

48

P Value Bashing

Every thinking physician, every thinking statistician, every thinking editor, and every thinking regulator has, at one point or another, had difficulty with the rigidity of *p* values. As physicians we learn to expect variability in our patients, and have developed a fine tool to deal with it—flexibility. We adjust treatment regimens if patients don't respond as anticipated. We alter testing schedules, increasing or decreasing the frequency of laboratory evaluations accordingly. We ask our colleagues to see our patients and we listen to their sometimes surprising advice. Flexibility serves us well in reacting to patient variability in our practices. However, it seems that statisticians respond to variability with staggering hyperrigidity. $p = 0.05$. If the p value is greater than 0.05 than "You missed it. What a shame. You worked so hard". If your p value is less than 0.05, then "Congratulations. Outstanding work. When will you publish?" How can we allow all of the work invested in a research program, all of the variability in investigators and in patients, all of the toil in collecting thousands of case report forms and hundreds of thousands of bits of information to be supercondensed down to one number? This is tremendous effort for one number which dispenses judgment on research programs (and—let's be honest—indirectly judges the quality of our efforts in those programs) unfeelingly, dispassionately granting publication acceptance, grant awards, academic progress, and regulatory approval. These p values seem to make or break careers and spirits, and it sometimes seems that we have no choice but to let them have their way.

It is perhaps only natural, given that the p value has so much influence, that we would expect investigators to reverse the tables by influencing them. Significance testing has been described as flexible and adaptable. Unfortunately, moves to utilize this flexibility and this adaptability have come at the expense of twisting the interpretation of p values. Every move toward flexibility has pulled p values farther from their intent and true meaning, distorting them.

Significance testing has become so problematic that some scientific journals are reacting with increasing vehemence against it. In 1987, for example, a dispute in the literature broke out when the prestigious and well-respected *American Journal of Public*

Health solicited an editorial which suggested point blank that significance testing be purged from articles submitted for review and
publication (significance testing reduced in significance, one could
say). The epidemiologist Alexander Walker debated with the statistician T.W. Fleiss, who, while supporting significance testing,
conceded that these same significance tests has been abused in
epidemiology and other fields [1–5]. He stated that readers often
equate statistically significant results with clinically significant
results. Fleiss also pointed out that insignificant effects are associated with negative studies, even though such studies have inadequate power and, can only be considered at best to be uninformative. However, Fleiss defended significance testing, saying
that it keeps us from coming to our own conclusions about the
results of an experiment, claiming that we need safeguards
against diversity of interpretation, imaginative theorizations, and
against the possibility that "my substantive difference may be
your trivial difference."

Is War Too Important to Be Left to the Generals?

Both the *p* value and the 0.05 rule have become preeminent—but
perhaps for the wrong reasons. Many readers have substituted the
0.05 judgment for their own thoughtful, critical review of the research study and critics of significance testing have concluded
that significance testing is synonymous with thoughtless decisions. Charles Poole [7] points out that the mechanical application
of a 0.05 (or any other arbitrary) decision rule requires no thought
and is therefore easy (once the decision rules have been set). He
is right in criticizing those who entertain the naïve hope that they
can find an easy way out of critical discussion in science by reflexively accepting *p* values. However, it would be wrong to conclude that thoughtless decisions must inescapably accompany significance testing.

Some have argued that significance testing is not an essential
part of statistics, and that epidemiologists and statisticians should
not be involved in decision making. Their job is to report and

tabulate the data and turn it over to others to make the difficult choices.[2]

Unfortunately, if we don't interpret the work, others will fill the vacuum. In 1998 it became law in Florida[3] to require that music by Beethoven be played for a segment of each day in every pre-school day-care facility. The genesis of this law is found with a powerful, influential Florida state legislator who came across a study that suggested that brainpower was increased in children exposed to this music. Never mind that the finding demonstrated only a transient increase in cognitive ability (twenty minutes). Never mind that this transient increase was never reproduced by other studies. The legislator believed exposure to Beethoven's music (eventually expanded to classical music in genenral) worked, and pushed the notion through the legislature to become state law. When asked about the dearth of supporting scientific data, the legislator responded "What harm can it do?" I for one would have felt much better if they had run the idea by an epi-demiologist or biostatistician. The French politician Georges Clemenceau said that "war is too important to be left to the gen-erals," but we cannot afford to let this paradigm characterize the role of statisticians and epidemiologists in research interpretation. Things may not be so great when statisticians and epidemiologists are involved, but disaster occurs when they are not.

Finding a Way Out

If we are interested only in the size of an effect (and its precision), with no need to make a single decision about the likelihood of that effect occurring in the population, then there is no need of a p value. Other tools, such as confidence intervals, can be em-ployed[4], and this is the tool to which some workers (particularly in epidemiology) have turned. However, if decisions must be made, then in concordant studies involving random sampling plans with important consideration given to the appropriate level of type I error, p values serve very well. If we must make deci-

---

[2] This is tantamount to the "Let Others Thrash It Out" discussion in the Prologue.

[3] Florida (Florida senate bill 0660 — signed into law 1998.

[4] Confidence intervals are discussed in chapter 4.

sions based on the data, the p value is our best option. Significance testing has been twisted by many, distorted by many others, and repudiated by some. However, just because p values are open to abuse and misuse does not mean they should be abandoned—we should simply insist that they be used properly—not as tools for thought evasion, but with appropriate reflection of the community standard for type I error consideration.

Less than the Sum of Its Parts

Statistics fulfills two roles, guiding the investigator as she examines the relationship between the presence of the risk factor and the occurrence of the disease. The first is to provide an estimate of the effect (e.g., a relative risk or an odds ratio, or a mean difference). This is termed *estimation*. The second is to help her infer what may be observed in the population based on the estimate she has in her sample. Often times, this inference focuses on the possible values of the effect size in the population.

This step of inference, of extending sample estimates to a larger population can be difficult, primarily due to sampling error. As we have seen in chapter 1, the investigator compromises by studying a sample of the population. By doing so, she acknowledges that she is unsure how accurately her sample represents the population at large, since the population can generate many samples each with different results. The tendency of a population with one effect size to produce different samples each with a different effect size (sampling variability), is very problematic when it comes to inferring from the findings of a sample back to the population. Significance testing is the traditional manner in which this sampling variability is taken into account. The researcher estimates the effect size in the sample using modeling tools, and then infers the findings of the sample back to the population. As defined in chapter 1, p values assess the probability that there is no effect in the population, but the population has produced a sample which contains a nonrepresentative effect. The smaller the p value, the more confident the investigator can be that the effect she has seen in her sample is due not to sampling error but to the correct reflection of a true population effect.

This distillation effort is perhaps at the root of the inappropriate role of significance testing. The supercondensation of the results of a research effort down to the p value may be due to the fact that the p value is itself constructed from several components. As we will see in the next section, an important ingredient in its construction is sample size. The size of the effect is also built into the p value. Finally, the precision of the effect size estimate (variability) is included. These three measures (sample size, effect size, and effect size precision) are all important ingredients that the investigator must consider when interpreting their research. However, their incorporation into the p value does not replace their consideration. The fact that these three measures of sample size, effect size, and effect size precision are embedded in the p value does not mean that research interpretation is equivalent to p value interpretation.

Actually, the p value is treated as being greater than the sum of its parts, when in fact it is less than the sum of its parts. Sample size, effect size, and effect size variability go into the p value. What comes out is not a balanced measure of these, but only a measure of the role of sampling error. Three ingredients go in, and one very different one emerges. Thus, p values are deficient by themselves, and must be supplemented with additional information (sample size, effect size, and effect size precision) in order for the study to have a fair and balanced interpretation.

This point requires reemphasis. P values receive important attention in applied statistics and epidemiology. However, they provide only an estimate of the role of sampling error in the research effort, nothing more. P values are not the repository of judgment for the study. P values do not measure effect size, nor do they convey the extent of study discordance. These other factors must be determined by a careful critical review of the research effort. Reflexively responding to p values as though they were the sum of all of their ingredients, when in fact they are less than that sum, often leads to inappropriate conclusions from research efforts.

Brief review of significance testing

The underlying thesis of research studies and hypothesis testing, is simply that those subjects who are treated differently, differ more than those subjects who are treated the same. Those who are treated the same have variability because of the inherent and natural differences between them. Those who are treated differently have this same natural variability plus the difference impose by the fact that some received an intervention, while others did not. Test statistics are constructed to identify and measure these two sources of variability. Most test statistics are ratios, the numerator containing the variability in the system due to a nonrandom effect (i.e., treatment effect) and the denominator reflecting the variability among those subjects who received the same treatment. Thus, the test statistic contains the effect size in the numerator, and the variability of the effect size in the denominator. If this ratio is large, we conclude more variability among those treated differently than those who received the same treatment, and, if the experiment was well designed and executed, we then attribute this excess variability to the treatment. Test statistics examine ratios of variability.[5] By converting the test statistic to a p value, the sampling error component is added.

Let's now leisurely work through a simple example of significance testing. A physician is practicing medicine in a community, seeing many patients with atherosclerotic disease. One of his roles is to help patients reduce thier LDL cholesterol levels, a task which often requires medication. The standard of care in his community is based on the observation that, in general, patients have LDL cholesterol levels less than 140 mg/dl and therefore most often need just one medication to reduce these values. Using this assumption, patients do not incur the cost of repeated cholesterol level determinations. Once the presence of atherosclerotic disease is determined the patient is placed on monotherapy. However, this investigator suspects that patients in the community he serves have LDL cholesterol levels greater than 140 mg/dl and wishes to draw a sample to assess this thesis. Such a finding would suggest to him that the single-therapy approach is not powerful enough, and that multiple medications would be required to reduce LDL-cholesterol levels. However, the investigator also knows that the use of these additional medications would be associated with an increased incidence of adverse effects in his

---

[5] When I was an undergraduate student, I could not understand why a test which had its null and alternative hypothesis stated in terms of means (of the difference between, say, the effect of different concentrations of an antibiotic on the growth of bacteria) was called "analysis of variance." This term was used by Fisher because the contruction of the test statistic is a ratio of variability due to the antibiotic (those treated differently) and the variance of those treated the same. The greater the variance, the more likely we are to believe the antibiotic caused the variability in treatment means, if designed appropriately.

community. He therefore wants to be sure that the data support the requirement of additional, more aggressive therapy before he advocates its use in the community. He plans to carry out a significance test to evaluate LDL cholesterol levels in his community. The investigator begins by selecting patients randomly from his community to determine LDL cholesterol levels. In order to reduce variability, he plans to have all of the LDL cholesterol levels measured by the same laboratory.

The underlying statistical reasoning driving this analysis is that the investigator knows that there will be variability in the LDL cholesterol levels in his sample of patients—different patients will have different cholesterol levels. In fact, he can plot this variability in a frequency distribution. The investigator believes that it is reasonable to assume that the LDL cholesterol levels in his community and in his sample will follow a normal distribution. If that is the case, then the mean LDL cholesterol level from his sample will be a very good estimator of the population mean LDL cholesterol level. Thus, if the sample mean is "far from" 140 mg/dl, the population mean LDL cholesterol level is likely to be far from 140 mg/dl as well.

Let μ be the unknown population mean LDL cholesterol level. We are now ready for the significance test, setting up the null and alternative hypotheses

$$H_0 : \mu = 140 \text{ vs. } H_a : \mu \neq 140$$

Now we must acknowledge here that the investigator does not believe the null hypothesis. If the investigator believed the mean LDL cholesterol level in his community was 140 mg/dl, he would continue advocating the current therapy regimen and would not bother with carrying out the research.[6] His clinical judgment and experience tell him that the alternative hypothesis is true. However the prevailing sense about his patients and their physicians, which he would like to disprove, is that the community mean LDL cholesterol is no greater than 140 mg/dl. He therefore must demonstrate to his critics the untenability of the null hypothesis, which represents that traditional and established view of LDL cholesterol levels in his community. The investigator does this by proceeding as though the null hypothesis is correct and that the community mean LDL cholesterol is 140 mg/dl. He takes a sam-

---

[6] Fisher called this the null hypothesis because it is the hypothesis to be nullified by the data.

ple of 225 patients with atherosclerotic disease randomly from his community. If the null hypothesis is true, he reasons that he would expect the mean of his sample to be close to 140 mg/dl. If it is not, then one of two possibilities must have occurred. The first is that the community "dealt him a bad hand," i.e., the community mean LDL cholesterol is 140 mg/dl but this population produced for him, just through the play of chance, a spurious sample with a sample mean LDL cholesterol far from 140 mg/dl. The probability of this outcome is the p value. However, the other possibility is that the null hypothesis is wrong, and the community mean is greater than 140 mg/dl, and the sample mean is close to the community mean. If the null hypothesis is wrong, it must be rejected in favor of the alternative hypothesis.[7]

Let's look at the alternative for a moment. It is stated as $H_a : \mu \neq 140$. This says that the community mean may be either less than 140 mg/dl or greater than 140 mg/dl. The investigator doesn't believe equally in each possibility. He believes the community mean LDL cholesterol is greater than 140 mg/dl. However, he doesn't know that it is (if he did, there would be no need for the experiment). Stating the alternative hypothesis as "$\neq$" appropriately separates his beliefs (he believes $\mu > 140$) from his imperfect knowledge (he really doesn't know where the community mean lies).[8]

Since an important component of this study is the sample mean, the investigator examines the sampling variability of this quantity (Figure 2.1).

Figure 2.1 reveals the theoretical frequency distributions of sample means from a normal distribution. The points of this curve may be considered to come from the following experiment. Take a sample of 225 patients and measure the mean LDL cholesterol. Then, take another sample of 225 patients, computing this sample's mean. Repeat this sample selection many times, each time computing the sample mean. Since the samples are each random samples from the same population, the degree to which these means vary one from the other is solely sampling variability. We see that the sampling variability permits the common occurrence of sample means from 138 to 142 to be produced from a community with a mean LDL cholesterol of 140 mg/dl.

---

[7] According to Fisher "Every experiment may be said to exist only in order to give the facts a chance of disproving the null hypothesis".

[8] One-tailed vs. two-tailed testing is the subject of chapter 6.

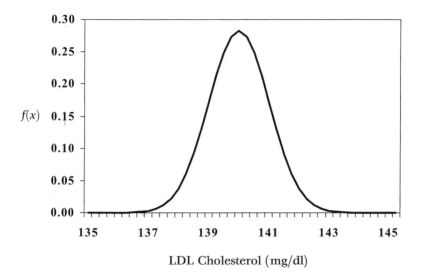

Figure 2.1. Probability distribution of sample mean LDL cholesterols: N = 225, $\sigma = 15$

However, what would we think if we observed a sample mean of 143 mg/dl? From an examination of figure 2.1 we would find that the occurrence of a sample mean as high as 143 mg/dl would be unlikely. Therefore, one way the investigator might proceed would be to conclude that the community mean is 140 mg/dl if he observed a sample with a mean LDL cholesterol less than 143 mg/dl. However, what if the sample mean was >143 mg/dl? The investigator could conclude that his sample was unrepresentative, but another reasonable conclusion is that the community mean is larger than 140 mg/dl.

In figure 2.2 the distribution of sample means is displayed for both the null hypothesis ($\mu = 140$mg/dl) and an alternate hypothesis ($\mu = 144$ mg/dl). These are the two possibilities the investigator would like to distinguish. Now he does not have the luxury of drawing many samples. He has only the time and resources to select and observe the results of one sample. The question is, when he has the mean from his one sample, how will he decide which of the hypotheses generated it? To guide him, he computes probabilities. For example, he could decide to reject the null hypothesis that $\mu = 140$ mg/dl if the sample mean is at least as large as 141 mg/dl. What is the probability that he would make the right decision? This is the probability that the sample mean is greater than or equal 141 mg/dl under the alternative hypothesis

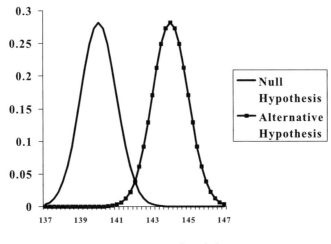

LDL Cholesterol Level (mg/dl)

Figure 2.2.   Probability Distribution of LDL cholesterol sample means under the under the null and alternative hypotheses: N = 225, $\sigma = 15$

that the community mean is 144 mg/dl or

$$= P[\bar{X} \geq 141 \,|\, H_a \text{ is true}] = P[\bar{X} \geq 141 \,|\, \mu = 144]$$

$$= P\left[\frac{\bar{X} - \mu}{\sigma_{\bar{x}}} \geq \frac{141 - 144}{1}\right] = P[Z \geq -3] \approx 1.00$$

which is reassuring, telling us that under the alternative, we might expect a sample mean as large or larger than 141 mg/dl virtually 100 percent of the time. Note that the numerator $\bar{X} - \mu$ is the effect size measure. The denominator $\sigma_{\bar{X}}$ contains the variability of the effect size, and also contains information about the size of the sample[9]. But, although the occurrence of a sample mean of 141 mg/dl or larger is a very common occurrence from a community with mean LDL cholesterol of 144 mg/dl, the investigator must also ask how likely would he expect a sample mean of 141 mg/dl or higher under the null hypothesis? He computes this analogously:

$$= P[\bar{X} \geq 141 \,|\, H_0 \text{ is true}] = P[\bar{X} \geq 141 \,|\, \mu = 140]$$

$$= P\left[\frac{\bar{X} - \mu}{\sigma_{\bar{x}}} \geq \frac{141 - 140}{1}\right] = P[Z \geq 1] = 0.159$$

[9] The variability of the sample mean $\sigma_{\bar{x}} = \sigma_X/\sqrt{n}$ where n is the sample size.

This is sobering. Although a sample mean of 141 mg/dl or higher is very likely under the alternative hypothesis, there remains a 16 percent chance that a community with a mean of 140 mg/dl will produce a sample with a sample mean of 141 mg/dl or greater.[10] If the investigator decides that the community mean LDL cholesterol is >140 mg/dl, he will launch a campaign to adjust the therapy regimens used to lower LDL cholesterol. This will mean the use multiple medications. The use of multiple medications will be associated with increased incidence of adverse effects in the community. Launching such a program based on a sample mean of 141 mg/dl implies a 16 percent chance that the community mean is not greater than 140 mg/dl and therefore the new program was unnecessary, and has harmed his community by exposing it to adverse effects in attaining an effect the community did not require. So, deciding in favor of the alternative for a decision at 141 mg/dl admits a 16 percent type I error.

Since this thought process is proceeding before the study begins, the investigator has the option of considering other decision rules. If the investigator chooses to reject the null hypothesis if the sample mean is greater than 141.96, the type I error is

$$= P[\bar{X} \geq 141.96 \,|\, H_0 \text{ is true}] = P[\bar{X} \geq 141.96 \,|\, \mu = 140]$$

$$= P\left[\frac{\bar{X} - \mu}{\sigma_{\bar{x}}} \geq \frac{141.96 - 140}{1}\right] = P[Z \geq 1.96] = .025$$

Consideration of the mirror image, that the community mean may be less than 140 mg/dl adds another 0.025 to alpha, bringing the total a *priori* alpha to 0.05. How likely is the occurrence of a sample mean greater than or equal to 141.96 under the alternative?

$$= P[\bar{X} \geq 141.96 \,|\, H_a \text{ is true}] = P[\bar{X} \geq 141.96 \,|\, \mu = 144]$$

$$= P\left[\frac{\bar{X} - \mu}{\sigma_{\bar{x}}} \geq \frac{141.96 - 144}{1}\right] = P[Z \geq -2.04] = 0.979$$

which assures us that the alternative hypothesis would commonly produce a sample with a mean LDL cholesterol >141.96 mg/dl.

The investigator now prospectively states the following decision rule: Reject the null hypothesis in favor of the alternative

---

[10] We are deliberately avoiding the complications of unknown variance and the use of a t distribution and other statsitical complications in order to stay focused on the underlying philosophy of significance testing.

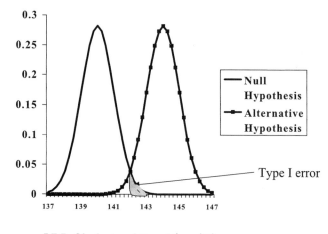

LDL Cholesterol Level (mg/dl)

Figure 2.3.   Probability Distribution of LDL cholesterol sample means under the under the null and alternative hypotheses: N $= 225$, $\sigma = 15$, $\frac{1}{2}$ type I error region denoted

hypothesis if the sample mean LDL cholesterol is more than 1.96 mg/dl from 140mg/dl.

The shaded area in figure 2.3 shows the portion of the critical region where the data are likely to be most revealing. Now the investigator has chosen his type I error at 0.05, distributing it across the two tails of the distribution. He has essentially told the community that he will advocate changing the LDL cholesterol reducing regime only if there was less than a 5 percent chance that he was misled by an unrepresentative sample. This is the prior alpha allocation. Note that this thought process proceeds before the first patient is accepted into the sample.

Now, finally, the study is carried out. Two hundred and twenty five patients are evaluated with lipid measures carefully obtained. The sample mean is 141.02, and the investigator carries out his significance test.

$$= P[\bar{X} \geq 141.92 \,|\, H_0 \text{ is true}] = P[\bar{X} \geq 141.92 \,|\, \mu = 140]$$

$$= P\left[\frac{\bar{X} - \mu}{\sigma_{\bar{x}}} \geq \frac{141.92 - 140}{1}\right] = P[Z \geq 1.92] = .027$$

and the two sided p value is $(2)(0.027) = 0.054$. The investigator has "just missed" the 0.05 level.

What happened? Are the results inconsistent with the investigator's concern that the community mean might have been 144 mg/dl? Under the alternative hypothesis,

$$= P[\bar{X} \geq 141.92 \,|\, H_a \text{ is true}] = P[\bar{X} \geq 141.92 \,|\, \mu = 144]$$

$$= P\left[\frac{\bar{X} - \mu}{\sigma_{\bar{x}}} \geq \frac{141.92 - 144}{1}\right] = P[Z \geq -2.08] = 0.981$$

It would be very reasonable that a sample with a mean of 141.92 or larger would be generated from a community with a mean of 144 mg/dl and, in fact, this close result would tempt some investigators to reject the null hypothesis. However, since it is also too likely that a community with a mean of 140 mg/dl would produce a sample mean of 141.92 mg/dl or larger we cannot discard the idea that the community mean LDL cholesterol value is 140 mg/dl or less. Since the p value is larger than his a priori alpha allocation of 0.05[11], the investigator concludes that the likelihood of a sampling error is too great. Based on his a priori decision, the risk of inappropriately treating the community is too high. Since the intervention has important side effects (some anticipated, some not), the decision provides protection for patients from unnecessary medications. The research program was successful, and community protection has predominated, i.e., concern for community protection militated against instituting a new therapy of marginal effectiveness. Also note how the effect size, variability of the effect size, sample size, and sampling error were incorporated into the p value. The p value is not an adequate measure for either of these first three, and should not be used as a substitute for them. The p value is not the sum of its parts. It is less than the sum of its parts, being an adequate measure of sampling error only.

Responsibilities and Mandates

In chapter one we spoke of the second preeminent responsibility of physician scientists—community protection. Every intervention has damaging side effects. Sometimes these side effects are anticipated; other times they are new and surprising. Medications are prescribed by physicians because these physicians believe

---

[11] Alpha levels are prospectively allocated—p values are measured experimentally, at the end of the study, and compared to the alpha set at the study's inception.

that the medicines, in balance, will do more good than harm. If the patients believe this as well, the side effects, with attention and treatment, will be tolerated. However, throughout this decision process, the physician must be assured that the medication will provide a benefit. Without this assurance, the patient is exposed to "medication" which is void of benefit, producing only side effects. This is the antithesis of "first do no harm," and the community requires protection from it.

This point is worthy of emphasis. Ineffective interventions in the medical community are not placebo—they are not harmless. Since medications have side effects, some of which can be severe, the physician must be convinced that substantial efficacy will be provided by the compound. The risk-benefit analysis physicians internalize presumes that there will be benefit. This assurance can be quantitated by physician investigators who fully accept their community responsibility.

The need for community protection is just as critical as the need for physicians to protect their patients. As physicians, we don't prescribe new drugs to patients who are already taking drugs without due consideration of the consequences. We start with lower doses, gradually escalating as needed. We monitor the patient frequently for evidence of side effects. These maneuvers are patient protective. However, since physicians can objectively view the effects of their therapy from sample based research, we must develop and maintain devices to protect the community from sample based errors. We anticipate the adverse effects. We are willing to run the risk these additional medications offer because of the drugs' proven effectiveness. We must have efficacy.

The demonstration of efficacy comes from clinical testing in clinical trials. Just as physicians must be vigilant about not using ineffective medications in their patients, the physician-scientists who execute these large experiments must be observant for lack of efficacy in the communities they study. In these trials, adequate protection must be provided for the community in which the drug is to be used. A type I error would could lead to the wide use of a drug whose efficacy was demonstrated in the sample studied but which has no efficacy in the community. Side effects are certain—efficacy is absent.

Physicians are in the decision making business and have an awesome responsibility. In order to make therapy decisions, they require a clear sense of the likelihood that the application of research results to the community will be different from those beneficial findings observed in the sample. Attaining this is an awesome task, but with that responsibility comes a mandate. This mandate requires the investigators to prospectively set the standard by which the study will be judged. Fortunately, the investigators are in the best position to do this. After all, they are often chosen for their scientific experience in general and their use of the intervention (e.g., a medication) in particular. They have expertise in administering the intervention, and are familiar with the intervention's dose-response relationship. The investigators use this experience to choose the study endpoints, ranking them in order of importance with great deliberation, marking them as primary or secondary. Investigators have strong conditions for choosing which patients will be admitted to the study (inclusion criteria) and which will not be permitted in the research (exclusion criteria). With such knowledge and experience, these physician-scientists have an in-depth appreciation of the intervention's strengths and weaknesses, yet, with all of this care and attention to details, they cede the community protection error level to a standard derived from agriculture.

Investigators have a mandate that they should use to set the a priori type I error level. By announcing their particular community protection responsibility prospectively, they appropriately set the terms of the post trial debate on the importance of the experiment's findings. However, in many studies, the investigators abrogate this community responsibility, acquiescing to the 0.05 standard.

Recall the LDL cholesterol level investigator of this chapter. Why did the researcher choose alpha of 0.05 here? If he chose it by tradition, I fear he made a grave mistake. The 0.05 level was based on agricultural intuition, and it would be useful to review what Fisher said about 0.05 (from the Prologue):

> For it is convenient to draw the line at about the level at which we can say 'Either there is something in the treatment or a coincidence has occurred such as does not occur more than once in twenty trials.' This level, which we may call the 5 per cent level point, would be indicated, though very roughly, by the greatest chance deviation observed in twenty successive trials.... Personally, the writer prefers to set the low standard of significance at the 5 per cent point, and ignore entirely all results which fail to reach this level".

The only way one can ignore results that fail to reach this level of 0.05 is to have good intuition about the poor reliability of such results when compared to the possibility that potentially promising results would be lost. Fisher said that anything above 0.05 should be ignored based on his intuition—the intuition of an agriculturist. There is no good reason at this point to dispute Fisher's choice of 0.05 for the prospective alpha statement for agriculture, but must it be applied to all fields of science? To medicine? To astronomy? To economic forecasting models? There is no unifying philosophical or mathematical theory that says all investigational science should have the same standard that was used in manure experiments seventy five years ago. New intuition must finally apply.

Investigators have good reason to carefully consider the prior alpha allocation level during the study's planning phase. In some circumstances, the 0.05 level is too restrictive. Consider the treatment of the unfortunate patients who are HIV positive. In the search to find effective treatment, we should leave no stone unturned and, as long as the study patients are well aware of the risks involved with the novel therapy, the investigations will be aggressive in the choice of therapy. Perhaps alpha levels as large as 0.25 are appropriate here, since we are willing to take the chance that the therapy may not work in the community at large, hoping that additional therapy based on this initial find will be developed and proven to be safe and effective in the end. Alternatively, there are circumstances where the 0.05 level is not stringent enough. For example, consider a disease for which the standard of care for a condition is well advanced, with patients having access to treatments which are effective and which produce few side effects, each of which are well recognized. In this case, any new therapy with a relatively unknown side effect profile[12] (and perhaps higher cost) must assure the medical community that the expensive switch to it will be worthwhile. In this setting, alpha levels on the order of 0.005 may serve us better than the reflexive 0.05.

The investigators have earned the right to freely choose the level themselves but they must do so prospectively, during the trial's inception. As investigators choose their alpha level, they will engage in discussions with members of the scientific com-

---

[12] The side effect profile will have been measured in the sample of patients studied; however, when used in a much larger population consisting of patients with comorbidities and other medications not used in the study, the side effect profile may appear much different.

munity, reaching a consensus on a range of appropriate alpha levels. One way to broaden this discussion is to write and publish a design manuscript. This is the statement of how the study will be conducted and how its data will be analyzed. Publication and promulgation of this document is a public statement, telling the community of the rules of conduct of the trial, and the standards chosen by the investigators to judge the trial as a success or a failure. Alpha levels must play a prominent role in such a manuscript if the investigators plan to draw conclusions about efficacy based on the sample data. If, at the study's end, the research effort is positive (i.e., the *p* value in the end is less than the alpha allocated in the beginning), the investigators must report the effect size and the *p* value. They should not hang their heads because the alpha allocation they chose a priori was different than that chosen by Fisher 75 years ago in a manure experiment.

Is there an alternative to *p* values?

The short answer is, if you are making dichotomous decisions (e.g., the therapy either works or does not work) no. If you are not making decisions, then there are several alternatives. One popular alternative is the confidence interval. This is the range of probable values of the population effect size based on the sample effect size and sampling variability. The greater the confidence interval's width, the less precision the estimator holds. However, some workers inappropriately make decisions about the strength of evidence an estimate contains based on whether the confidence interval contains the value of the estimator under the null hypothesis. This easy transformation of a confidence interval into a "back-door hypothesis test" (i.e. if the range of values covers the value of the parameter under the null hypothesis then $p > 0.05$), should be avoided. If you are going to carry out significance testing, then carry it out. Prospectively state your intention, frankly and explicitly execute the test, and report the result.[13]

Another possibility is the use of a likelihood function as advocated by Allen Bernbaum [8]. Likelihood functions provide graphic evidence of the data's strength of support for candidate

---

[13] Some advice on p value interpretation in observational studies where the exposure cannot be randomly allocated is offered in chapter 3.

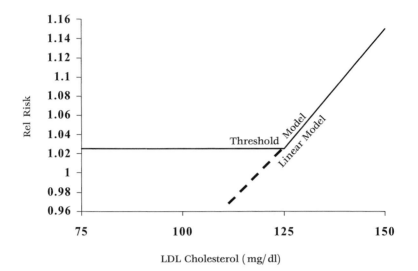

Figure 2.4.   Post Randomization LDL Cholesterol—Event Relationship

values of the population parameter of interest. An example of a
likelihood function would be as follows. In the ongoing debate
concerning LDL cholesterol reduction in secondary prevention
(i.e., in patients who already have a history of atherosclerotic cardiovascular disease). Several studies (CARE, LIPID, and 4S) have
demonstrated that these patients benefit from cholesterol reduction therapy. The question is, how low can a patient's LDL cholesterol level be driven before there is no further benefit? Several
research groups argue that the relationship between LDL cholesterol and the occurrence of events is linear—the lower the LDL
cholesterol, the lower the risk of morbidity (figure 2.4). Other
groups argue for a threshold effect in LDL reduction. The group
that argues for a threshold effect must identify the hinge point in
the LDL event relationship, i.e., at what level of LDL cholesterol
does the slope of the LDL cholesterol—event curve change?

Identifying the hinge or threshold at which the slope of the line
changes can be extremely problematic. A single hypothesis test
that is "all or none" for an a priori specified hinge point can be
limiting. What is useful here is a depiction of the likelihood function.

Figure 2.5 depicts the likelihood of candidate LDL cholesterol
values as the hinge point. The x-axis represents the candidate
values for LDL, and the "height" of the graph reflects the data
set's support for that LDL value being the hinge point. The graph

Candidate LDL cholesterols

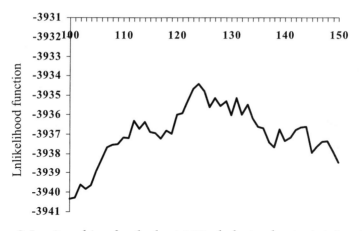

Figure 2.5. Searching for the best LDL cholesterol cutpoint. Log Likelihood by LDL cholesterol

suggests that there is data support for a hinge point at 124–125 mg/dl. Although there does appear to be a peak in the function here, there are alternative candidate points, none of which is far from 125 mg/dl. In this complicated situation, a likelihood function evaluation provides additional information (interpreted in an exploratory light) not conveyed in hypothesis testing. Even a confidence interval approach would fail to convey the unevenness with which the data support various alternative hinge points.

We should now return to the morose investigator with whom we introduced this chapter. With all of the work the investigator invested in the design of the trial, he in all likelihood did not give much thought to the 0.05 standard. There is no theoretical justification for 0.05 and, in fact, the 0.05 level is absolutely arbitrary. Explicit consideration of the current standard of care for the population would most certainly have led to another level. The investigator would have been better served by thinking through the implications of sampling error, and choosing his own alpha level independent of the Fisher standard. These conversations would no doubt have been both interesting and rewarding. If this investigator's effort did not reach the prespecified 0.05 level, then at least he could say that, although the research effort was promising, protection standards that he tailor made and custom fit for the community of interest prohibited this study from being interpreted as positive. That's not a bad message. Now, all he can say is that his research is not positive because it did not reach a goal in whose construction he did not participate and whose relevance he does not understand.

Conclusions

Statistics can never yield scientific truth" claimed the nineteenth century physiologist Claude Bernard. He argued that in order for medicine to be treated as a science, its knowledge must be "based only on certainty ... not on probability". Both the critics and the advocates of significance testing recognize that sampling variability will require statistics to stay firmly embedded in medical research.

The p value provides an estimate of the role of sampling error in our research efforts, nothing more. P values are not the repository of judgment for the study. P values do not measure effect size, nor do they convey the extent of study discordance. They do not measure the extend of confounding. These other factors must be determined by a careful, critical review of the research effort. Reflexively responding to p values is shortsighted thought evasion. Frankly, if you want to let p values do your thinking for you, it's probably time that you get out of this business.

We cannot conclude that just because we see a small p value, that p value is the product of a meaningful experiment. In fact, in these disputatious times, it is incumbent on the investigator to persuade us that the study is relevant, measures an effect of interest, can be generalized to the population, and is a fair appraisal of how the results are influenced by biases in the study. If she cannot convince us in each of these matters, the p value should provide no solace for her. P values cannot rescue discordant studies, and small p values do not cover a host of methodological sins.

We must also acknowledge that the Fisher 0.05 standard has become the accepted standard, for no reason other than tradition. Although this is accepted practice, it is time for us to say that this is bad practice. Later in this book, we will see its inadequacy for more complicated research programs with multiple treatment arms and multiple endpoints not envisioned by Fisher. In these complicated experimental environments, alpha must certainly be controlled but, to interpret these experiments usefully, we must discard the tradition of 0.05, instead bringing our mandate as investigators to bear in order to set the alpha levels intelligently and prospectively. Children grow out of their clothes. The old clothes may be familiar and may contain fond memories, but they no longer fit. We have grown beyond 0.05. We have paid homage long enough. It's time to turn our backs on the shrine.

References

1. Walker, A.M., (1986) "Significance tests represent consensus a and standard practice," *American Journal of Public Health* 76:1033. (See also Journal erratum 76:1087).
2. Fleiss, J.L., (1986) "Significance tests have a role in epidemiologic research, reactions to A.M. Walker," *American Journal of Public Health* 76:559–560.
3. Fleiss, J.L., (1986) "Confidence intervals vs. significance tests: quantitative interpretation," *American Journal of Public Health* 76:587.
4. Fleiss, J.L., (1986) "Dr. Fleiss response," *American Journal of Public Health* 76:1033–1034.
5. Walker, A.M., (1986) "Reporting the results of epidemiologic studies," *American Journal of Public Health* 76:556–558.
6. Lang, J.M., Rothman, K.L., and Cann C.L. "That confounded p value," *Epidemiology* 9:7–8.
7. Poole, C., (1987) "Beyond confidence interval," *American Journal of Public Health* 77:195–199.
8. Bernbaum, A., (1962) "On the foundations of statistical inference," *Journal of the American Statistical Association* 57:269–326.

3

Mistaken Identity: *P* Values in Epidemiology

Mistaken Identity

On the eve of one of his battle campaigns, the emperor Napoleon took the time one evening to make an unannounced, personal inspection of his army. During this inspection, while he walked from unit to unit, he came across a guard who had fallen asleep at his post. The leader shook the dozing soldier awake, demanding to know his name so that the guard could be officially reprimanded. The guard replied smartly, "Sir, my name is Napoleon", to which the enraged emperor replied "Sir, either change your character or change your name!"

The *p* value is a foot soldier mistaken for an emperor. It is falsely considered by many to be all that one needs to know about a research study's results. Perhaps this is because incorporated within the *p* value are many of the measures that everyone agrees are necessary for a balanced interpretation of concordant research programs. The *p* value construction explicitly considers and includes sample size, effect size, effect size variability, and sampling error. Each of these components is important in the interpretation of a study. Since the *p* value encapsulates these, it is easy to see why many could believe that the *p* value is the sum (and perhaps greater than the sum) of its parts.

This "sum of the parts" philosophy has perhaps been one of the contributors to the *p* value's preeminence in research, but is fallacious, and epidemiologists have been quite vocal in their recognition of this problem of mistaken identity. The experience of epidemiologists with observational (nonrandomized) studies has motivated them to fight to topple the p value from its position of preeminence. However, we will see that the p value itself, with its "sampling error only" interpretation, is not the problem and that a disciplined, well-circumscribed, sampling-error perspective on the p value permits it continued use by health care researchers.

Detective Work

Epidemiology is the scientific discipline that focuses on the research methodology used to identify the cause and effect relationships in health. Traditionally, epidemiology has been associated with the identification of the cause of disease (e.g., the identification of polluted water sources as the cause of gastrointestinal illness in London) and with the identification of effective treatment for a disease (e.g., the role of citrus fruit ingestion in the prevention of scurvy). Through skillful use of observational research methods and logical thought, epidemiologists work to assess the strength of the links between risk factors and disease.

Epidemiologists speak not so much of intervention, but of exposure (exposure to benzene, exposure to diet pills, etc.) in nonrandomized research efforts. The term "nonrandomized" refers to the lack of random allocation of the intervention. In these research efforts, it is not logistically or ethically feasible to randomly assign patients to exposure. Without the tool of random therapy (or here, exposure) allocation, attribution of the effect size seen in the research program can become complicated.

I sometimes think of my epidemiology colleagues as the good detectives who get only the toughest cases to solve. Many important studies and landmark research efforts (e.g. the Framingham analyses) have been nonrandomized. These studies have been, and will continue to be, critical. What is the relationship between the heavy metal content of tooth fillings and the occurrence of disease in later life? What is the relationship between silicone breast implants and autoimmune disorders? The relationship between magnetic field exposure and cancer in children? The relationship between prescription diet pills and valvular heart disease? Unfortunately, in each of these circumstances, although it can be easier to select candidates randomly from the population at large, it is impossible to randomly allocate the exposure among subjects in the sample. Nevertheless, the answers to the exposure-disease relationship in each of these studies are critical. By and large, public health has advanced on the backs of nonrandomized studies and the epidemiologists who design, execute, and analyze them. But, as the examples earlier in this paragraph demonstrate, the role of randomization in these studies is by necessity restricted, and, *p* values, unless carefully interpreted are less helpful when perhaps their sharpest interpretation is most needed.

Definition of Causation

A central issue in health care research is the ascertainment of the true nature of a relationship. Risk factors and disease can be related in one of two different ways. An *association* between a risk factors and disease is the observation that the risk factor and the disease simultaneously occur in an individual. Causal relationships on the other hand are much stronger. A relationship is *causal* if the presence of the risk factor produces the disease in an individual. The causitive risk factor *excites the development* of the disease. This causal relationship is tight and contains an embedded directionality (i.e., the risk factor was first present in the absence of the disease, then the risk factor excited the production of the disease). The declaration that a relationship is causal has a deeper meaning then the mere statement that a risk factor and disease are associated. This deeper meaning and its implications for health care require that the demonstration of a causal relationship rise to a higher standard than just the causal observation of the risk factor and disease's joint occurrence.

Determining Causation

Just as justice is more than simply reciting from a book of laws, the determination that a risk factor—disease relationship is causal requires more than the blind application of artificial rules. Risk factor—disease relationships are unique and each require specific attention. For example, there are circumstances in which a strong risk factor—disease relationship first reported as suggestive of causation was subsequently shown to be non-causative and coincidental. On the other hand, there are clear examples of risk factor—disease relationships identified by a single examination of a series of cases which are clearly causative. Two of the clearest examples of this are the link between thalidomide and birth defects, convincingly detected Lenz [1]. and the Seldane-Ketoconazole link with deadly irregular heart beats [2]. In each of these cases, one and only one study was required to demonstrate causality. Furthermore, each was a case series on a case report. The most important lesson one can take from this is that the determination of causality is a thinking person's business. There is no substitute for clear observation, deliberative thought, and careful deductive reasoning in consideration of the true nature of a risk factor—disease relationship.

Experimental vs. Observational Studies

We should begin by distinguishing between experimental and observational studies. In an experimental study, the investigator has control over the intervention or exposure assignment. He controls the choice, timing, dose, and duration of the intervention whose impact he wishes to measure. In observational studies, the researcher does not provide the intervention, choosing instead to observe the already existing patterns in the link between the occurrence of the risk factor and patients with the disease. We may divide experiments into two categories of experiments; randomized vs. nonrandomized experiments. In randomized experiments, the selection of the intervention is not based on any characteristic of the subjects, insuring that the only difference between subjects who receive the intervention and those who do not is the intervention itself. Thus, when a difference in the endpoint measure between intervention groups is identified at the end of the study, that difference can be ascribed or attributed to the intervention.[1]

---

[1] Randomization is the best tool to reduce confounding in experimental design.

Randomization

Randomization is the hallmark of modern experiments. We have seen that it is an adaptation that received considerable attention from Fisher's early work (see prologue), and, although its appropriateness in clinical experiments is still debated, it has had a major impact on the development of medical science. Generally in clinical experiments, there are two levels of randomization. The first is the random selection of subjects from the population, a concept discussed in chapter 1. The second is the random allocation of the experimental intervention. Each has a different goal and follows a different procedure. It is desirable in clinical studies to utilize the random selection of subjects, and if an intervention is involved,[2] to incorporate the random allocation of this intervention as well.

As we have discussed in chapter 1, the random selection of subjects from the population at large implies that not just every subject in the population has an opportunity to be accepted into the study, but that every subject has the same, constant probability of being selected. This simple random sampling approach is the best way to insure that the obtained sample represents the population at large, and that the findings in the sample can be generalized to the population from which the sample was obtained. Whenever random sampling does not take place, broad generalizations from the sample to the population at large are often impossible. However, it is also true that this level of randomization creates in the sample the property of statistical independence, which allows for the multiplication of probabilities so useful in the construction of both parameter estimators and test statistics.

There is a second level of randomization, however, which is critical in many research efforts. The random allocation of therapy, when present, occurs within the selected sample itself. This procedure insures that each subject in the sample has the same, constant probability of receiving the intervention, effectively prohibiting any link between the intervention and characteristics of the subjects themselves. The presence of this level of randomization is crucial for the clearest attribution of effect to the interven-

---

[2] The presence of an intervention whose allocation the investigator controls is the hallmark of an experimental study, as opposed to an observational study, where the investigator observes relationships already in place in the sample.

tion. Once the investigator identifies an effect in the sample, he wants to attribute that effect to something. In an experiment, the investigator wishes to attribute the effect to the intervention he has assigned in the experiment. If the only difference between patients who receive the intervention and those who received a control is the intervention (the percentage of males is the same across groups, the age distribution is the same across groups, the race distribution is the same across groups, etc.), then differences in the outcome measure of the experiment (e.g., mortality) can be ascribed to the intervention. The absence of the random allocation of therapy in an experiment clouds the attribution of therapy effect. In an extreme case, if all patients who receive the active medication happened to be women and all who receive the control happened to be men, it is impossible to determine if the difference in outcome measure should be attributed to the intervention or to gender.[3] The random allocation of therapy is a design feature that, when embedded in an experiment, leads to the clearest attribution of that therapy's effect.

Large clinical trials attempt to take advantage of both of these levels of randomization. Undoubtedly, the researcher conducting the experiments have little difficulty incorporating the random allocation of the experimental intervention. Proven randomization algorithms are required to be in place at the trial's beginning, assuring that every patient who is accepted into the trial sample must have their treatment randomly allocated. In addition, once researchers randomize patients, examinations of baseline characteristics in each of the randomized groups are thoroughly reviewed, insuring that demographic characteristics, morbidity characteristics, and results of laboratory assays are distributed equally across the two groups. These procedures and safeguards work to insure that the only difference between subjects who receive the intervention and subjects who do not is the intervention itself. The treatment groups are the same with respect to all other characteristics, traits, and measures.

It is difficult to overestimate the importance of randomization. Use of this tool not only protects the experiment from the influences of factors that are known to influence the outcome, but it also protects against influences not known to affect the occurrence of the endpoint, again because the random assignment of

---

[3] We say that the effect of therapy is confounded (or confused) with the effect of sex.

therapy does not depend on any characteristic of the individuals. When randomization fails to correct for a variable such as age, there are some techniques that can correct the analysis for differences caused by age. However, in randomized experiments, adjusted results will rarely differ markedly from unadjusted results.

Unfortunately, the random selection of subjects from the population in these randomized clinical trials is not guaranteed. It is true that large clinical experiments randomize patients from many different clinical centers. These centers represent different regions of a country, different countries on a continent, and sometimes different continents. This widespread recruitment effort is an attempt to be as inclusive as possible, and the investigators hope that it results in an acceptable approximation of this random selection mechanism.

One impediment to the random selection of subjects from the population in these large clinical studies is the use of exclusion criteria. Patients who are intolerant of the intervention cannot be included in the study. Patients who are in other studies cannot be included. Patients who have life threatening illnesses are often excluded as well.[4] Patients who are unlikely to be able to follow the compliance criteria of the experiment (patients who cannot take the intervention consistently or patients who refuse to adhere to a tight schedule of followup visits) are often excluded as well. These exclusion criteria are often necessary for the successful execution of the trial, but they certainly weaken any argument that the experiment has followed a simple random sampling plan. Thus, although large clinical trials successfully randomly allocate therapy, they are not so successful in the random selection of subjects from the population.

Observational studies, as opposed to experimental studies, are research efforts in which the investigator does not introduce an intervention but observes relationships that are already in place in the sample. Observational studies are sometimes termed "epidemiologic studies." This is somewhat of a misnomer, since the interpretation of all research programs (be they experiments or not) invoke epidemiologic principles, but remains a communicative distinction based on tradition.

---

[4] An unfortunate patient who has terminal pancreatic cancer with less than one year to live is unlikely to be randomized to a five-year trial assessing the role of cholesterol reduction therapy in reducing the number of heart attacks, even if they have met all other criteria for the trial.

Nonrandomized, observational studies can sometimes do a better job than their counterpart clinical trials in randomly selecting subjects from the population. Although these observational studies are rarely able to randomly allocate exposure in their attempt to assess the relationship between exposure and disease, they nevertheless play a critical role in the development of public health. These studies are often (but not always) less expensive and administratively easier than their randomized trial counterparts. Most often these complicated studies fall within the purview of epidemiologists.

Collisions

"Since the study found a statistically significant relative risk ... the causal relationship was considered established[3]."

What a statement! Most every biometrician and epidemiologist would disagree with it on face value. However, the very fact that it could be made suggest how far afield significance testing has gone. P value interpretations in epidemiologic studies often lead to head-on collisions between biostatisticians and epidemiologists. Biostatisticians, with their emphasis on the computational assumptions of the test statistic and the long term accuracy of the p value[5] tend to emphasize their use. Epidemiologists tend to discount p values in these observational studies, primarily because of (1) their realization that p values have bound up (confounded) in them information about sample size and effect size, and (2) their inability to clearly interpret p values because of the absence of randomization of the exposure.

The fiery significance testing debate flared up with a 1998 editorial in *Epidemiology* entitled "That Confounded p value[4]" in which the editors argued that the p value has bound up within it the influences of sample size and effect size. Such built in tension in one number purported to be a summary of a research effort, the editors argued, cannot be allowed to be influential in assessing scientific endeavors. *Epidemiology* has chosen to expunge p values "in any context in which confounded elements can be

---

[5] The long term accuracy of the p value is a concept emphasized by statisticians who subscribe to the frequentist interpretation of statistics, and is discussed in chapter 10.

conveyed conveniently, either numerically, graphically, or otherwise." At first, it may seem like the editors, in their vehemence, are acting much like the architect who, dissatisfied with the final physical appearance of the home he has designed, rather than fire all of the workmen, instead bans them from using hammers. Such a policy of *p* value exclusion forces the reader to disentangle exposure or treatment effects from background sampling variability — something the reader needs help with, not direct exposure to.

This confusion is unfortunate, and perhaps has at its center a case of mistaken identity. These astute editors are correct. *P* values *do* have a host of influences built into them, including sample size and effect size. However, *p* values were not designed to convey this information but only to state the degree to which sampling error affects sample based decisions — nothing more. *P* values must be jointly interpreted with each of sample size, effect size, and effect size precision (e.g., confidence interval or standard error) for the researcher to gain a balanced perspective of the study's results. The clearest interpretation of the study (not the *p* value, but the study) also requires the random allocation of exposure; difficulty with attribution of effect circumscribes the conclusions in nonrandomized designs. Realization of these limits of *p* values has led to their rejection by many epidemiologists — and if these workers see *p* values as summarizing a research study's conclusion, then they are correct in rejecting this interpretation. However, *p* values can be of importance as long as they are seen as statements solely about sampling. When considering *p* values in any study, observational or experimental, they must be relegated to statements about sampling error.

Strengths and Weaknesses of Different Research Designs as Contributors to the Tenets of Causality

Causality is the principal relationship of interest in epidemiology. The assessment of whether an attribute or characteristic is the direct cause of a disease and not merely associated with it is a question which is asked very easily, but often answered with great difficulty. The databases coming from the researchers on a particular exposure-disease relationship are complicated, and the arguments raised by opposing sides of the causality argument can be complex. This data collection is often teeming with associations and relationships that are sometimes surprising, sometimes not. Sometimes these relationships are due to sampling error, and sometimes not. The application of the causality tenets helps to distill this information down to a compact body of knowledge, governed by a few master principles. In their work, epidemiologists often link statistical considerations with other observational ingredients necessary to build a strong causative argument between an exposure and a disease.

Tenets of Causality

It is important to note that an in-depth mathematical background is not required in order to understand and appreciate these tenets. Although mathematical sophistication is sometimes necessary to assess the contribution a research effort makes to the tenet, the tenets themselves and an understanding of how they form the building blocks of a causality argument require no deep understanding of mathematics.

The principles rest on the insight that follows from sharpened powers of observation and deductive reasoning. Bradford Hill [5] suggested that the following aspects of an association be considered in attempting to distinguish causal from non-causal associations:

1. Strength of Association
2. Consistency
3. Specificity
4. Temporality
5. Biologic Plausibility
6. Gradient or Dose Response
7. Coherence
8. Experimental Evidence
9. Analogy

A brief description of each follows.

Tenet 1:   Strength of Association
Strength of association is the magnitude of the effect of the exposure on the prevalence of the disease. In observational studies,

this is most often the odds ratio or the relative risk. Epidemiologists commonly report this measure with a confidence interval, which provides some estimate of the precision of the effect size. The narrower the confidence interval, the greater the precision of the estimate. *P* values are sometimes used here, and can be of some value if the investigators and the readers can dissociate *p* values interpretations from sample size, effect size, effect size variability, and effect attribution.

Tenet 2:   Consistency

The persuasive argument for causality is built much more clearly on a collection of studies, involving different patients and different protocols, each of which identifies the same relationship between risk factor exposure and effect. The numerous studies, with different designs and patient populations, that have identified the same hazardous relationship between cigarette smoking and poor health outcomes is a clear example. The disparate results from studies examining the impact of silicone breast impact and autoimmune disease make it difficult to argue (at least on this single tenet) for a causality relationship.

Tenet 3:   Specificity

The greater the number of possible causes, the more difficult it becomes to identify a single cause for the effect. Malignant pleural mesothelioma has asbestos exposure as its one principle cause. Multifactorial diseases, e.g., atherosclerotic cardiovascular diseases, have a host of causes (e.g. elevated lipids, elevated blood pressure, cigarette smoking, diabetes). It is difficult to identify an additional cause because the established ones may influence the new "cause."

Tenet 4:   Temporality

The presence of the risk factor must precede the event for which it is hypothesized to cause. Occurring after the exposure is not synonymous with being caused by the exposure (*post hoc ergo proctor hoc*) but it is a necessary condition. This may seem like a simple concept, but can be vexatious to verify. It is best explored by explicitly building the correct timing relationship into the research design. Without appropriate attention to this condition, protopathic bias (drawing a conclusion about causation when the effect precedes the risk factor in occurrence) can result.

Tenet 5: Biologic Plausibility

It is easiest to accept an association between exposure and disease if there is some basis in scientific theory that supports such a relationship. The scientific community is more likely to believe a relationship between levels of serum lipids and heart disease because of the extensive research carried out to elucidate the relationship between lipid deposits and endothelial pathophysiology. However, a relationship between the birth month of a patient and the occurrence of heart attacks is implausible, as there is no discernable mechanism that would explain the relationship between these two variables. However, the issue of biologic plausibility is tightly linked to the maturity of our understanding of the pathophysiology of the disease progress.

Tenet 6: Gradient or Dose-Response

This tenet focuses on the presence of a graded relationship between the causative agent and the effect. An example would be the observation that the higher a patient's diastolic blood pressure, the greater that patient's risk of stroke. This gradient response makes it much less likely that an extraneous factor related to both the risk factor and the disease are related is an explanation of the underlying risk factor—disease relationship. Dose response therefore represents an important demonstration of the influence of the causative agent on the disease.

Tenet 7: Coherency

This implies that a cause-and-effect interpretation for an association does not conflict with what is known of the natural history and biology of the disease.

Tenet 8: Experimental Evidence

If the exposure has been associated with the occurrence of disease, can removal of the exposure be linked to a decrease in the incidence of the disease? Such an experiment would add greatly to the strength of evidence for a causality argument. Challenge-dechallenge-rechallenge studies are especially useful in satisfying this criteria.

Tenet 9: Analogy

Establishing a link between a risk factor and disease can be aided by a related link having been understood and accepted in the base. For example, it is somewhat easier to link drug use during pregnancy with the occurrence of congenital defects when the scientific community already accepts as a useful, previous example the existence of a causal link between thalidomide use and congenital abnormalities.

Epidemiologic Research Designs and Problematic P Values

We have seen the criteria used to determine the presence of a cause-effect relationship. In order to demonstrate these tenets, epidemiologists have embedded structure into observational research design to demonstrate these tenets while maintaining the ability to efficiently work with data in several constructs. The result has been a collection of different research designs, each with the ability to satisfy some of the nine Bradford Hill causality tenets. An assessment of the strength of a causal argument comes from as assessment of the entire body of knowledge, oftentimes consisting of several observational studies of different designs. The job of the reviewer is to synthesize the total research effort, determining which of the causality tenets each of the research studies has satisfied.

In working to construct a body of evidence, epidemiologists are rarely able to turn to tools of randomization. It is not that they reject the notion, only that they do not have the luxury of being able to design a research effort will include randomization of exposure. In addition, there are ethical issues here, since many would argue that it is not ethical to execute a research program involving the random assignment of an intervention believed to be harmful. Ethical concerns precluded the execution of such randomized experiments, yet information on the risk factor— health outcome relationship is required to enact effective public policy. Over the course of scientific research, several alternative nonrandomized investigative designs have evolved. It is useful to consider the nomenclature and the distinguishing features of these designs, keeping the focus on the correct interpretation of *p* values. As long as the *p* value is relegated to a statement concerning sampling error, it is relevant in epidemiologic studies.

Directionality: Looking Forward or Looking Backward

Directionality refers to the type of inference between the risk factor and disease in a research program's effort and determines the condition of the relationship between the risk factor and the disease. The program can either have a forward inference (risk factor presence implies disease prevalence) or a backward inference (disease status implies exposure). The concept of directionality is separate from the retrospective vs. prospective concept that we will describe momentarily.

To demonstrate the directionality characteristic in clinical research, let's consider two observational study designs evaluating the relationships between coffee ingestion and pancreatic cancer. The first investigator identifies patients with pancreatic cancer (cases), say in a registry or in a review of hospital records. He then identifies patients who do not have pancreatic cancer (controls), derived from the same population as his cases. After this determination of cases and controls, the researcher looks into the history of these patients to determine their coffee ingestion history. The investigator then identifies the proportion of the cases who had exposure to coffee, and computes the proportion of the controls who had coffee exposure. The research question asked here is, given a patient has pancreatic cancer, how much more likely is the patient to have ingested coffee? This is a backward inference, moving from case identification back through time to prior coffee exposure.

The second investigator starts by collecting not cases based on the presence of cancer but with cancer-free individuals who drink coffee. She identifies patients from the same population who do not ingest coffee. She follows her exposed and unexposed group forward through time, to determine the incidence of pancreatic cancer. This would be a forward study, since first the exposure's presence is assessed and then, for patients with the exposure and those without, the occurrence of the endpoint is measured. The research question is how much more likely is pancreatic cancer in those who drink coffee than in those who do not. This is a forward inference and can be easier for the nonepidemiologist to understand.

Both of these designs addresses the coffee ingestion-pancreatic cancer issue, but from different directions. The first (backward approach) moves from the case identification to the exposure. The second (forward approach) begins with the exposure and moves to identify disease. Determining the criteria on which the cohort is assembled is the hallmark of directionality. If identified by exposure status, the design is forward; if identified by case status, the design is backward.

If one remembers that the p value reports only sampling error and not attribution of effect, the p value may provide some useful information. However, in neither of these two designs was coffee exposure randomly allocated, and the researcher must always be clear that the p value says nothing about whether the pancreatic cancer is due to the exposure as opposed to something confounded with the exposure. The p value interpretation is straightforward if we keep this distinction in mind. Sample size and effect size, along with a measure of the effect size variability must also be reported. However, since the coffee exposure was not assigned randomly, reporting the four features of sample size, effect size, effect size precision, and the p value itself do not completely clarify the study's interpretation, since the researcher could not be sure that the difference in the occurrence of pancreatic cancer was specifically due to the coffee ingestion.[6]

Typically, when the case prevalence is rare, forward direction studies will require many more patients than backward studies, since the forward study must identify a large number of exposed and unexposed patients to collect an adequate number of cases. For the backward study, since the cohort is selected first based on cases, attention is focused on first identifying an adequate number of cases matching them to controls, and ascertaining exposure on this relatively small cohort.

Timing — Retrospective vs. Prospective

Timing can be retrospective, cross-sectional, or prospective. Unlike directionality, which addresses the characteristic on which the cohort was chosen, timing asks whether the information was collected in the past, or will be collected in the future. When did

---

[6] For example, the panceatic cancer could have been due to cigarette smoking, dietary habits, exercise habits, each of whch may itself be related themselves to coffee exposure. Adjusted analyses, discussed later in this chapter, can help to reduce difficulties in effect attribution.

the risk factor and disease onset occur? If these occurred before the research was undertaken, and we must gather this information reflecting only past events, our research is completely retrospective. If the study factor ascertainment will occur in the future, and the disease onset occurs in the future, we have a completely prospective design.

In a retrospective study, the researcher uses information that has been collected from the patient in the past. Thus, the researcher is compelled to review records about the patients' past experiences. The investigator identifies the information about exposure from subject recall, from previous medical records, even from autopsy and postmortem toxicology information. To identify disease status, he again identifies the past occurrence of disease, and it totally dependent on what information was available in the past. In retrospective studies, the design is held captive by the abundance or dearth of this historical data.

Prospective designs allow the researcher more flexibility. Not being limited to past information, the researchers can tailor the collection process to the research program, fortifying the ability of their effort to identify the risk factor—disease relationship. In a prospective design, the researcher has the opportunity to collect the information about the patient's current condition directly from the patient, with little reliance on recall. The investigator can choose to collect information in the level of detail that is necessary, rather than settling for what is available in a retrospective research program. Thus, in a prospective program the data can be collected to address more subtle issues in the exposure disease relationship, often making the research program more convincing. For example, the researcher can choose to measure different levels of exposure that would allow an examination of the dose-response relationship in the research program. Also, if randomization of exposure cannot be implemented, the researcher can collect information that is known to be correlated with either exposure or case prevalence, allowing a more convincing covariate adjusted analysis.

Each of the features of directionality and timing can be used to help understand the following types of observational studies that are most useful to investigators.

Case Control Studies

Subjects are identified as having an event (e.g., a stroke). Patients who do not have the event (controls) are then chosen. The history of each case and control is then searched to determine if the patient has the risk factor (e.g., hypertension). The investigator hopes to show that patients with stroke are more likely to have hypertension than are patients without stroke. However, this is not equivalent to demonstrating that patients with hypertension are more likely to have a stroke than are patients without hypertension. In a sense, the passage of time is backwards, i.e., first identify cases and controls, then go back to see if the patient had the risk factor. For these reasons, classic case control studies have a backward directionality.

Cross-Sectional Studies

In these studies, both exposure and disease status are measured simultaneously. Thus, these research programs are nondirectional; they involve no passage of time. However, since this design provides no sense of time, the timing criteria of the tenets of causality cannot be assessed. For example, a cross-sectional study can identify the prevalence of cardiac arrhythmias in patients on antiarrhythmic agents, but it cannot determine if those agents change the occurrence of these heart rhythms.

Prospective Cohort Studies

These studies can be very persuasive, since they first identify the risk factor, then follow the patients forward (prospectively) to determine if the endpoints (e.g., heart attacks) occur. However, they are not experimental since the investigator does not assign the risk factor, and therefore the attribution of effect can be problematic. Consider a research program designed to measure the relationship between homocysteine levels and the occurrence of heart attacks. Researchers measure patients' homocysteine levels and then follow them for three years to assess the incidence rate of myocardial infarction (heart attack). It is possible to link the incidence of myocardial infarction to the presence of depressed levels of homocysteine. However, since there may be many of the differences between patients with low and high homocysteine levels that may not be known and therefore cannot be adjusted for, this study cannot successfully attribute differences in myocardial infarction to differences in homocysteine levels.

Historical Cohort Studies

The historical cohort study is an example of a retrospective, forward design. It is related to a prospective cohort study, but it is "run in the past." For example, in the homocysteine level–heart attack study described as a prospective, cohort study, the investigators observe homocysteine levels now, then follow patients into the future to determine which of them sustain heart attacks. Suppose instead that this study was carried out in an established, complete database. The investigator first looks back into the early segment of the database to determine each patient's homocysteine level, and then looks forward in the database to determine the occurrence of heart attacks. This is like a cohort study embedded in retrospectively collected data. Since it is retrospective, it contains the additional problem of being unable to correct for differences in the groups not already available in the database.

Adjustment of Variables in Observational Studies

We have pointed out that, in observational studies, there is no random allocation of exposure, with consequent difficulty in effect attribution. Regression analysis is sometimes used to correct observational studies by adjusting for differences between the exposed and unexposed groups.[7] Many argue persuasively that this adjustment is more important in observational studies, since in these studies there is no random allocation of the risk factor of interest, and that there are differences between exposed and in-exposed patients that confound our ability to ascribe an effect to the risk factor of interest. These adjustments may go a long way in reducing the problem with effect attribution in observational studies. By reducing the influence of known confounders on the exposure-disease relationship, the attribution of effect becomes clearer. However, adjustments are not as effective as randomization and must not be seen as an adequate replacement. One can correct an observational study for the effect of age using regression analysis, but that correction does not remove all of the imbalances between the risk factor and non- risk factor groups. In fact, an investigator can correct for all known differences between the risk factor and non-risk factor groups through the use of re-

[7] Regression analysis and p value interpretation are discussed in chapter 9.

gression analysis. However, because the investigator can correct
only for known risk factors (assuming he has the values of these
risk factors in the dataset) and unknown factors may be determining the differences between the two groups, he will never
fully get the exposed groups and unexposed groups statistically
equivalent. In the random design, however, the use of the random allocation assures the investigator of equivalence between
the intervention and nonintervention groups[8]. Adjusted analyses
are very useful, but cannot replace the random allocation of exposure.

The use of the procedure of adjustments through regression
analysis can help to clarify the attribution of effect. However, the
light shed by the *p* value remains the same. It illuminates only
sampling error. Even in adjusted analyses, *p* values must be
interpreted jointly with sample size, effect size, and effect size
variability.

Design Considerations

The goal of research efforts is often to examine the relationship
between a possible risk factor for a disease and the occurrence of
the disease. We have seen here that scientists have a range of
study designs at their command to investigate this question. Each
of these types of study designs provides important information.
However, there is a relationship between the cost (financial cost,
logistical cost, patient cost) and ethical considerations of that
study, and the type of information each study provides about the
risk factor—disease relationship.

Many consider, prospectively designed, double-blind clinical
trials to be the state-of-the-art investigational tool of clinical investigators. The (approximate) random selection of subjects from
the population and random allocation of therapy allow for the
clear attribution of therapy effect. However, the cost of selecting a
large number of patients from the population at large, controlling
the intervention, and following patients prospectively over time
for years is often prohibitively expensive. The retrospective prev-

---

[8] The use of randomization may fail for an isolated variable, but once the adjustment is made using regression analysis, the groups are equivalent since the randomization procedure all but assures equivalence on all other risk factors.

alence study is an alternative design that provides important data on the relationship between a risk factor and a disease. Because they involve carefully choosing the level of exposure to observe and methodologically measuring the occurrence of the disease, these prevalence studies provide important information on the relationship between the risk factor and disease. These studies not only conserve financial resources—they conserve patient and administrative resources as well.

However, the price one must sometimes pay for these cost-effective retrospective studies is the potential distortion of the risk factor-disease prevalence relationship through the operation of biases (e.g., selection bias, recall bias, and ascertainment bias, to name just a few). Thus, researchers must balance the relatively weaker causality arguments developed from the cost-effective retrospective studies against the stronger causality evidence from the prohibitively expensive prospective randomized trials. In weighing the relative advantages and disadvantages of these different designs, scientists have reached a consensus. Like a tool in a tool kit, each design has a set of circumstances to which it is uniquely suited. In the first investigation of a rare disorder, there often are not the financial resources or the groundswell of support from the public health community for a large-scale, prospective clinical experiment. In this circumstance, the researcher will reach for the retrospective, observational study. Easily designed and relatively inexpensive, it will efficiently capture and quantify the magnitude of the relationship between the risk factor and the disease. If the strength of the relationship (the signal) is strong enough to overcome the methodological biases that can sometimes blur or distort this signal, enthusiasm grows for carrying out more expensive experiments.

The causality tenets are the filter through which each of the research efforts is poured. This filter traps the limits and weaknesses of the designs, and executions. What is left is the strength of evidence for a causal relationship between exposure and the disease. When applying the causality tenets, one would like to identify a growing body of evidence that contributes to the strength of association. For example, in the investigation of the relationship between cholesterol levels and ischemic heart disease, the first observations of cases were followed by case control studies, and then by studies that examined the effects of cholesterol levels on a population (ecological studies). These were then followed by case studies that demonstrated the reduction in the incidence of heart attacks by cholesterol reducing therapy, again through case studies, and then by observational studies(Framingham). These studies were followed by randomized controlled clinical trials (WOSCOPS, 4S, CARE, LIPID).

Regardless of which research design is implored, the p value must have a tightly circumscribed sampling error interpretation. In concordant, observational studies where effect attribution can be difficult, as well as in concordant clinical trials that employ the random allocation of therapy, the study interpretation must include explicit consideration of each of the p value, sample size, effect size, and effect size variability.

Solid Structures from Imperfect Bricks

The demonstration of a causal relationship between a risk factor and a disease is complex. The assessment of this relationship cannot and must not be viewed solely from the perspective of a randomized controlled clinical trial, and the point of view that randomized controlled clinical trials are necessary for causality must be carefully considered. The reflexive refusal to recognize a causality relationship solely because of the absence of a randomized clinical trial is dangerously close to "thought avoidance" and must be shunned. There has been no randomized clinical trial to demonstrate the asbestos exposure-pulmonary disease link, yet advocates of clinical trials have not called for a trial that randomizes (i.e., chooses at random) patients to receive a deliberate for heavy asbestos exposure in order to demonstrate the harm asbestos can cause. There has been no randomized clinical trial to demonstrate the hazards of ingesting foul, soiled water, yet the hazard has been made amply clear, justifying important community standards for fresh, healthy water. There have been no randomized clinical trials to demonstrate the hazards of smoking—any attempt would be correctly seen as flagrantly unethical—yet the hazards of smoking are amply apparent. Clearly, randomized clinical trials are not necessary to demonstrate causation.

Observational studies are not randomized, yet they can be so well designed and executed that they become the kernel around which a persuasive body of knowledge for a cause and effect relationship crystallizes. In 1998, the federal Food and Drug Administration (F. D. A.) has removed terfenadine (Seldane) from the market due to evidence of an undesirable effect of the combined used of seldane and some antibiotics. This decision was made not based on a clinical trial, but based instead on compelling data from case report information and from observational studies. Mebifridil (Posicor) was removed from the marketplace by the F. D. A in 1998 in the presence of compelling information from case series reports in the face of equivocal evidence from a clinical trial. In each case, the information for causality was satisfied by information from nonrandomized research efforts. Clearly, there is ample precedent for deciding causality in the absence of a randomized controlled clinical trial.

The collection of such studies, each of which examines the risk factor−disease relationship must be considered as the body of evidence. No study, not even the gold standard, randomized clinical trial is perfect. Nevertheless, buildings of sound and solid constitution can be constructed from imperfect bricks. In the end, it is the final edifice which must be judged.

How to Draw Inferences From Epidemiologic Studies

It cannot be overstated that, although the p value must be carefully evaluated in nonrandomized studies, these studies can still be designed and executed skillfully to provide important, unambiguous evidence for causality. Epidemiologists recognize that the nonrandom nature of the most commonly used designs does not preclude them from building a strong argument for effect size in the population. Epidemiologists build inferential arguments by the following these guidelines.

1 − Choose the sample with care.
A nonrandom sample does not mean a careless sample. If the epidemiologists are choosing cases and controls, they must insure that patients who are cases and controls come from the same population. If they are choosing exposed patients and unexposed patients, they must insure that these exposed and unexposed patients come from the same population.

2—Use the tool of matching judiciously.
Matching insures that an effect size in the end cannot be due to
the matched variable (e.g. sex or treating physician), since the
distribution of the matched variable is the same between cases
and controls. It is a useful tool in clarifying effect attribution.

3—Execute the effort concordantly
Although it is a maxim that well-designed research is prospectively
designed research, a necessary corollary is that the research must
be well executed, minimizing protocol deviations. This concordant
execution allows a clear separation between prospectively planned
analyses, and exploratory analyses.[9]

4—Report sample size, effect size, confidence intervals and p value.
Each of sample size, effect size, confidence intervals and *p* value
provides important information. The information from each of
these sources is not independent. Sample size information is incorporated into effect size measures, and sample size, effect size,
and effect size variability are incorporated into the *p* value. The
clearest assessment of the strength of association is consideration of the information from all four sources. The interpretation should include joint examination of these measures of the
experiment.

5—Rely on adjusted analyses
Regression analysis is a necessary procedure in observational
studies, since they have no random allocation of the risk factor of
interest, and there are differences between the group with the risk
factor and the group without. This adjustment is carried out by
first isolating, and then identifying the relationship between first,
the covariate and exposure, and second, between the covariate
and the disease occurrence.[10] These relationships are removed
before the assessment is made. These corrections, provided as
adjusted odds ratios or adjusted relative risks, are important ingredients of epidemiologic studies, which attempt to clarify the
attribution of the effect to the risk factor. Such adjustments are
not essential when exposure can be randomly allocated, but, in

---

[9] Exploratory analyses not stated prospectively have no prior alpha allocation,
and are executed post hoc and cannot be used as a formal test of a statistical
hypothesis. These are discussed in chapter 10.
[10] There is a more complete discussion of adjusted analysis in chapter 8.

observational studies, adjustments insure that the results cannot be explained by differences in known risk factors for the disease, and add greatly to the clarity of effect attribution. Adjusted analyses, although they do not replace the random allocation of therapy are a very useful tool in epidemiology.

Study counting: The ceteris parabus fallacy

Study counting is simply counting the number of studies that address a risk—factor disease relationship and deciding if there "are enough" studies to support the notion that the risk factor causes the disease. Some who are involved in study counting argue that there must be more than one study. Others say that the number of positive studies must outnumber the number of negative studies. Only the fortunately rare and rarely fortunate epidemiologist reduces the argument of causality to "study counting". Instead, the scientific reasoning process assesses in detail each of the available studies, carefully dissecting the methodology, sifting through the patient characteristics, and methodically considering the conclusions. Study counting represents the wholesale abandonment of the intellectual principles of careful consideration. In a word, study counting is scientific thoughtlessness and should be rejected as a tool of inquiry.

This point requires a more detailed examination. The specific problem with "study counting" is the implicit *ceteris parabus* (all other things being equal) assumption, i.e. that all of the studies which are being included in the count are equal in methodology, equal in the thoroughness of their design, equal in the rigor of their execution, and equal in the discipline of their analyses and interpretation. This fallacious assumption is far from the truth of scientific discovery. Studies have different strengths and different weaknesses. Different investigators with their own non-uniform standards of discipline execute the research efforts. Some studies give precise results, while others are rife with imprecision. The panoply of studies is known not for their homogeneity, but for the heterogeneity of designs and interpretations.

We must distinquish between the appearance of an *isolated* study, i.e. one study whose finding was contrary to a large body of knowledge available in the literature, and the occurrence of a sole study. There is ample epidemiologic evidence that single studies, when well designed and well executed can be used to prove causality (e.g. the thalidomide investigation). What determines the robustness of a research conclusion is not the number of studies but the strength and standing of the available studies, however many there are. Science, like the courts, does not *count* evidence—it *weighs* evidence. This is a critical and germane distinction. Study counting turns a blind eye to study heterogeneity. Our business in science is to think—not to codify thoughtlessness.

Critiquing Experimental Designs

A valuable skill of health care workers who review research efforts is critically reviewing the design, execution, and analysis of a research effort. This ability is essential to sifting through the weight of evidence for or against a scientific point of view and comes only with practice.

To start, begin with the realization that the successful critique of an experiment does not end with, but begins with a list of that research effort's strengths and weaknesses. The best critiques (you should not begin a critique unless it is going to be a good one; a poor one is a waste of your time) converts the catalogue of strengths and weaknesses into an argument for accepting or rejecting the findings of the research.

A useful approach to the critique of a research effort is as follows. Start with a review of the hypothesis and goals of the research effort. Then, before proceeding with the actual methodology, turn away from the manuscript and begin to construct for yourself how you would address the hypothesis. Assume in your plan that you have unlimited financial resources, unlimited personnel resources, and unlimited patient resources. Think carefully and compose the best research design, the design that builds the most objective platform from which to view the results. Only after you have assembled this design yourself should you return to read the methodology, the results, and the actual interpretation of the research effort that was executed. Having constructed your own "virtual" state-of-the-art design, you can easily see the differences between your design and the one that was actually executed by the researchers. After identifying these differences, ask yourself whether and how the compromises made by the researchers limit the findings of the research effort. It they pose no limitations when compared to your design, the researchers did a fine job by your standards. If the researchers have substantial limitations, then the analysis and its generalizability may be crippled. The researchers may have had understandable reasons for the limitations, but these limitations can nevertheless undermine the strength of their findings.

Conclusions

Epidemiologic studies have been the cornerstone of the development of public health research programs and continue to make important scientific contributions to public health understanding and policy. Unfortunately, the nature of these programs often precludes the random allocation of exposure.

P values have a rich history of use in observational studies, and although, at one time they were embraced, p values have fallen into some disrepute. The difficulty with p values in these important, nonrandomized efforts is that they have erroneously but commonly been interpreted as binding up the truth of the trial—sample size, effect size, sample variability and effect attribution—into one number. Workers who interpret p values in any research study, imbuing them with interpretative powers beyond an assessment of sampling variability, unfortunately do so at their own risk. The situation is more acute in nonrandomized studies due to the absence of the random allocation of exposure in the sample chosen from the population. P values can play a useful role in the causality debate if the researchers are clear that p values were not designed to measure sample size, effect size or effect attribution, only sampling error.

References

1. Lentz, W., (1962) "Thalidomide and congenital abnormalities," (Letter to the Editor), *The Lancet* 1:45
2. Monahan, B.P., Ferguson, C.L., Kileavy, E.S., Llyod, B.K., Troy, J., Cantilena, L.R., (1990) "Torsades de Pointes occurring in association

with terfenadine use," *Journal of the American Medical Association* 264:2788–2790.

3. Anonymous, (1988) "Evidence of cause and effect relationship in major epidemiologic study disputed by judge," *Epidemiology Monitor* 9:1.

4. Greenland, S., (1990) "Randomization, Statistics, and Causal Inference," *Epidemiology* 1:421–429.

5. Rothman, J.K., (1990) "Statistics in nonrandomized studies," *Epidemiology* 6:417–418.

6. Hill, B.A., (1965) "The environment and disease: association or causation?" *Proceedings of the Royal Society of Medicine* 58:295–300.

7. Sacks, F.M., Pfeffer, M.A., Moye, L.A., Rouleau, J.L., Rutherford, J.D., Cole, T.G., Brown, L., Warnica, J.W., Arnold, J.M.O., Wun, C.C., Davis, B.R., and Braunwald E., (1996) (For the Cholesterol and recurrent Events Trial Investigators). "The effect of pravastatin on coronary events after myocardial infarction in patients with average cholesterol levels," *N Engl J Med* 335:1001–1009.

4
CHAPTER

Loud Messengers— *P* Values and Effect Size

Part of the application process for medical school admissions includes an interview with several faculty at the institution. While visiting one medical school that was considering me as a candidate, I was interviewed by a basic scientist—a neurophysiologist. During our conversation, the topic eventually turned to research. The interviewer finally commented that he was lamenting over a failed manuscript submission. Indulging my request for additional information, he related that his manuscript had been rejected by a prestigious journal, apparently for lack of statistical significance. Since I had some exposure to *p* values, we discussed their meaning and nonmeaning, jointly groping toward some inner truth, and finally realized together that "statistical significance" does not go hand in hand with clinical significance. We together broke some of the bonds with which *p* values had tied us so tightly. The purpose of this chapter is to break some more.

In the previous chapter we discussed the difficulty with interpreting observational studies, determining that the *p* value retains some value if the researchers remember that *p* values provide information only about the degree to which sampling error affects the results. *P* values convey nothing about sample size, effect size, or effect attribution. In randomized controlled clinical trials, these limitations also apply. In particular, the *p* value provides little unbiased information about the magnitude of the effect size. Small *p* values can be associated with very small effects as well. The *p* value cannot be relied on to convey effect size information. We must keep focused on the fact that what we are really after is the magnitude of the effect. The *p* value is just a way to measure one possibility for the meaning of the effect size observed in the population (which is that the effect size may actually be zero in the population). There are other parts of the effect size that the *p* value does not measure. A *p* value is like an uninformed messenger. The messenger may arrive with much noise and fanfare, yet when we open the package he delivered, we find that it is of no real importance. On the other hand, the the *p* value may be large, (or the *p* value may be absent altogether) yet the results can be of cataclysmic importance. *P* values can be small and yet measure effects of no real value. *P* values can be large, yet identify a signal in the data which cannot be ignored. In some research circumstances, *p* values add no tangible value to the finding.

P values and Effect sizes—the LRC Trial

Clinical trial results are often described in terms of the *p* value as though the *p* value alone conveys the strength of evidence of the findings. However, when a small *p* value is identified with a small effect size the findings can be of limited usefulness. This occurred with the Lipid Research Clinics study which was designed to demonstrated that the sustained reduction of cholesterol would lower the incidence of fatal and nonfatal heart attacks. In order to demonstrate this, the researchers selected 3810 men between the ages of 39 and 59 years of age, with total cholesterol levels greater than 265 mg/dl from the population at large and randomize them to receive either cholesterol-reducing therapy or placebo. The investigators interpreted this trial as positive with a *p* value <0.05.[1] The seven year cumulative incidence of fatal and nonfatal heart attacks was 8.6 percent in the placebo group and 7.0 percent in the active group, a reduction of 19 percent. This seems impressive, but what was the clinical significance of the findings? A quick computation revealed that one hundred men would have to be treated for seven years in order to avoid one fatal or nonfatal heart attack, at a cost of $12,000 per patient [1]. Actually, no one

---

[1] The reasoning behind this interpretation is provided in chapter 6.

really knew what to do what that number at the time[2], although this treatment appeared to be very expensive treatment relative to its clinical effect. This was one of the first trials that had anything like a cost- effectiveness computation carried out. The p value was small, suggesting much promise, yet the clinical effect remained a modest one.

This is the difference between clinical significance and statistical significance (related through the p value). In a well-designed, concordantly executed experiment, the p value can provide useful information concerning the role sampling error may have played in the study's results. However, clinical significance is quite another matter. Clinical significance has more to do with the impact of the findings on the community being treated. Clinical significance addresses whether there is a big enough payoff for the therapy. Additional, thoughtful examinations of the data must be relied upon to provide this information, the p value does not convey it.

Measures of Effect Size

We may examine the role of clinical significance in nonrandomized epidemiologic studies as well. There are several measures of effect size, each of which can convey important information. One useful one is the notion of odds. In general, the notion of odds used in biostatistics is consistent with the notion held by the public. The odds of failure represent how many more times an event will lead to failure then to success. For example, we say that when a coin which is fair is flipped, the odds of it landing on heads are 1:1 or even odds for a head. If the coin is twice as likely to be a heads than as a tail, we say that the odds of getting a "heads" are 2:1. Odds ratios are the ratio of two values, one occurring in a different set of circumstances (e.g. exposure vs. nonexposure). In general, the larger the odds ratio between the exposure and the disease, the stronger the degree of association between the two.

A note of caution must be sounded however. First, the odds ratio computed from the ratio of odds as observed in the sample.

---

[2] This occurred before the dominance of managed care with their cost effective treatment algorithms.

To what degree does this reflect the exposure of disease in the population? It is a certainty that another investigator will have collected a different sample of patients and obtain different odds ratios. Which is correct? Sampling error concerns remain important. Also, the anticipated lack of randomization of exposure complicates these studies' interpretation.

Consider the issue of the popular anorexigens or diet drugs fenflurmine/dexfenfluramine. Under pressure from the Federal Food and Drug Administration (F.D.A.) the manufacturer removed this compound from the market in September 1997, because of the association between its use and either primary pulmonary hypertension (PPH) or heart valve disease. Establishing a causal link with either of these conditions can be difficult. PPH is a disease where the blood pressure in the vessels from the heart to the lungs is very high. It is a different disease from essential hypertension or high blood pressure, which has received so much attention in the media and at doctors' offices. High blood pressure is a very prevalent condition that, after many years, is associated with the occurrence of heart disease, stroke, and kidney disease. It is easily treated with readily available medications, some of which have been shown to improve survival in patients with high blood pressure. PPH is an entirely different clinical entity. Unlike high blood pressure, PPH is very rare (with an approximate annual incidence rate of 1 to 2 patients per one million.) Unlike high blood pressure, PPH is very difficult to diagnose. No blood pressure measurements that can be taken in a clinic that provide useful information about the occurrence of PPH. Oftentimes, PPH is diagnosed only after the patient is in right heart failure, with difficulty breathing, fatigue, swollen, tender abdomen and liver, and swollen extremities. There is no good treatment for PPH. Unlike high blood pressure, PPH can kill patients after an acute, short-lived shock-like episode, or cause fatal heart failure after only three to four years of symptoms. PPH is rare, hidden, lethal, and difficult to treat, and must not be confused with systemic high blood pressure.

If every patient who was exposed to diet drugs subsequently developed PPH, and every patient who was not exposed to diet drugs did not, the task of measuring the strength of association would be very easy. However, in reality, there are patients who are exposed to anorexigens who do not develop PPH. This fact may make us think that exposure to diet drugs is not so dangerous. On the other hand, some patients who have no exposure to

Table 4.1. Relationship Between Exposure to diet drugs and Primary
Pulmonary Hypertension Prevalence

	Exposed	Unexposed	Total
Cases of PPH	30	65	95
Controls	26	329	355
Total	56	394	450

diet drugs will get PPH, since anorexigens are not associated with
all cases of PPH. The presence of such cases weakens the association of diet drugs and PPH, and the absence of such cases
strengthens the association. How many of these cases are too
many? To guide them, epidemiologists turn to elementary mathematics to quantitate the strength of association.

Consider the following examination of the relationship between
exposure to diet drugs and the prevalence of PPH, taken from
Aberhaim's[3] study and displayed in Table 4.1.

We will use these findings to simply compute some measures
of association. There are several elementary probabilities to compute here. The first is the probability of exposure, given that the
patient has contracted PPH which is $30/95 = 0.316$. The probability that the patient was not exposed, given that the patient contracted the disease is $65/95 = 0.684$. The odds that a patient with
PPH was exposed to diet drugs is just the ratio of these two numbers $0.316/0.684 = 0.462$. Approximately 32 percent of patients
with PPH were exposed to diet drugs (perhaps in combination
with other agents, perhaps not), while 68 percent of cases had no
known exposure. However, we need to know the experience of
those patients who did not have PPH in order to develop a more
complete picture of the anorexigen-PPH relationship. The computations for the controls are as follows. The probability that a
patient who is a control is exposed to diet drugs is $26/355 = 0.073$
while the probability that a patient is unexposed is $329/355 =$
0.927. Already we see that the probability of exposure for a case
(0.316) is greater than the probability of exposure for a control
(0.073). We continue by first computing the odds for exposure
when the patient is a control: $0.073/0.927 = 0.079$. The odds
ratio (OR) of exposure for cases to controls is $0.462/0.079 =$
5.85, indicating that the likelihood of exposure is almost six times
greater for cases than for controls. The magnitude of the odds ratio

---

[3] The numbers on which the following computations are based are taken from
Lucien Abenheim [2].

(OR) provides the strength of association. When the disease prevalence is low, as with PPH, the odds ratio approximates the relative risk.

Computation of the odds ratio factors in the background disease prevalence. Another useful quantity is the attributable risk (AR). This is merely the difference in the odds between cases and controls. In the case of Table 4.1 the AR = 0.462 − 0.079 = 0.383. Yet another useful computation is attributable risk exposed (ARE). This is obtained by subtracting one from the odds ratio, and then dividing this difference by the odds ratio itself. Being equivalent to the(odds(exposed)−odds(unexposed))/odds(exposed), this is the percent increase in disease prevalence that is attributable to the exposure. In this example ARE = (0.462 − 0.079)/0.462 = 0.83. This is commonly interpreted to mean that there is an 83 percent chance that the exposure has produced an increased risk of PPH. A better interpretation would be that in the sample, 83 percent of the increased prevalence of PPH in those exposed to diet drugs is due to that exposure. One other interpretation is that 83 percent of the cases of disease in those exposed would not have occurred if the exposure had been absent.

These computations of attributable risk exposed serve as the foundation for the rule that an odds ratio of two demonstrates sufficient strength of association, a rule sometimes used in legal arguments involving causation.[4].The attributable risk exposed for patients with an odds ratio of 2 is (2 − 1)/2 = 0.50, interpreted to mean that 50 percent of the excess prevalence of the disease among the exposed was due to exposure. The conclusion that 50 percent attributable risk exposed is large enough for public action is supported by Oullet [3]. In a study of attributable deaths due to smoking, for example, Oullet et. al. the researchers found 18 percent of all Canadian deaths were due to smoking and hazardous drinking (i.e., attributable risk exposed = 0.18). The authors described this attributable risk as large and further stated that this result was of considerable importance to policy makers. They also noted that successful actions or strategies directed towards these two factors could prevent a sizeable proportion of the premature mortality in Canada. Finally, an attributable risk exposed of 0.50, although large, does not imply that say that there is a 50 percent chance that the exposure caused the disease, for, as we have seen,

[4] Further elaboration on legal consideration is provided later in this chapter.

the other tenets of causality (timing, gradient, plausibility, consistency, etc.) are additional necessary ingredients for causality. Odds ratios, attributable risk, and attributable risk exposed address only the single criterion of strength of association.

Confidence Intervals

Although the computations above are useful, we know that they are based on just one sample. Since the population can generate many different samples, each including different patients with different histories and therefore different odds ratios (as well as different attributable risk, and different attributable risk exposed) how do we know that the ones generated from our own sample are correct?

The honest answer is that we don't know, but we can use the information from our one sample to generate a range of odds ratios that may be most reflective of the population odds ratio. Continuing the example from Table 4.1, epidemiologists convert the odds ratio of 5.85 into a range of odds ratios which would express the relationship in the population. A confidence interval is the range of candidate odds ratios in the population that would produce a sample with an odds ratio of 5.85. Computations for odds ratios are based on a "percent confident" basis. A 95 percent confidence interval is a range of candidate odds ratios for the population in which we are 95 percent certain that the true population odds ratio lies. The "95 percent" part of this is interpreted as follows. Say we had not just one sample, but 100 samples, and from each sample, generated a 95 percent confidence interval. We now have 100 confidence intervals. The true population odds ratio would be contained in 95 of these 100 intervals. This is it. We don't know which of the 95 intervals contain the true odds ratio, but we hope that our sample's 95 percent confidence interval will contain the true OR. Elementary mathematics (which we will not demonstrate here) leads to the computation of the odds ratios confidence interval 3.25 to 10.54 from Table 4.1 Note that this confidence interval contains the estimate of the odds ratio 5.85. We can compute an approximate range of attributable risk exposed in this computation of from 0.69 to 0.91. The correct interpretation of this interval is that we are reasonably assured that in the population, between 69 percent and 91 percent of the excess occurrence of PPH in those exposed to diet drugs is due to diet drug exposure.

Backdoor Significance Testing

The larger the odds ratio, the stronger the association between the exposure and the disease. However, the odds ratio should be precisely measured. Some have argued that if the confidence interval for an odds ratio contains the number 1, then the findings of the sample are inconsistent with exposure being associated with disease. However, because of the pesky problem of sampling variability. We must discard this notion which at first seems so direct and comforting, primarily. It is true that the confidence interval is the range of odds ratios that may reflect the exposure-disease relationship in the population, based on the sample taken from the population. If the measure of the odds ratio is precise, then an odds ratio of one says that the odds of exposure when the disease is present is the same as the odds of exposure when the disease is absent. This implies that there is no association between disease and exposure. It is a common mistake to hasten to a conclusion concerning the confidence interval without making a statement about the variability of the estimate around which the confidence interval was built. A wide confidence interval is a clue that the odds ratio estimate from the sample is imprecise. If the confidence interval contains one but is wide, then our estimate of the odds ratio is too imprecise for us to draw a conclusion. In fact, the odds ratio may be much greater than one, but its true value may have been masked by the sampling variability. This situation is akin to attempting to listen to a song on the radio when there is a great deal of background noise and static; so much that you cannot hear the song. Since all you were able to hear was the noise, you may want to conclude that there was no song to be heard. In fact, the song was there, but you missed it in all of the static. Just because you didn't hear the song doesn't mean that the song wasn't played. The signal of a large confidence interval can be lost in the background noise of sampling variability. All you can really conclude is that the entire exercise was frustrating and uninformative.

Also, we must admit that the confidence interval generation is related to significance testing. The value 1 contained in the odds ratio confidence interval is synonymous with a two sided p value greater than 0.05. We have already demonstrated that significance testing must be tightly circumscribed and allowed to contribute only to arguments concerning sampling errors. Furthermore, it is unwise to pluck one value from a confidence interval and draw a conclusion about the population odds ratio. Many have criticized this practice in the epidemiologic literature, most notably WD Thompson [4] and Poole [5]. As Poole discusses, rejecting the extreme values of a confidence interval simply because it includes the value 1 discards valuable information about the population and should be rejected. He deplores the inconsistent double action of workers who generate confidence intervals then draw conclusions as though a significance test had been carried out. We might term this improper use of a confidence interval as a "back-door significance test."

Both Thompson and Poole suggest that attention must be paid to the bounds of the confidence interval and not merely to whether the confidence interval contains the value 1. Thompson points out that values just outside the confidence interval are only slightly less likely to occur than are values in the confidence interval. In making an assessment of what values of the odds ratio are supported by the population, it is prudent for the worker to consider the potential benefit and hazards to the population in drawing a conclusion. If an approximate confidence interval for attributable risk exposed contains two, then it is quite possible that the attributable risk exposed for the population is at least 50 percent, much greater than the 18 percent identified in the study of Ouellet for excess mortality in Canada due to smoking and alcohol ingestion.

Clinical Significance Without *P* Values

In the previous example, p values were not invoked. In some cases, they are not even necessary. Has there been an epidemiologic study that assessed causality in the absence of multiple studies with minimal reliance on p values? Yes.

The drug thalidomide has a long FDA history [6] Thalidomide was hailed as a "wonder drug" that provided a "safe, sound sleep." It was a sedative that was found to be effective when given to pregnant women to combat many of the symptoms associated with morning sickness. No one suspected that the drug, whose name became synonymous with terrible adverse effects would cross over from the bloodstream of the mother to that of the unborn baby until it was too late.

Thalidomide was synthesized in West Germany in 1954 by Chemie Grünenthal and introduced to the market in the 1950s. It was approved in Europe in 1957, and marketed from 1958 to 1962, in approximately forty-six countries under many different brand names. A U.S. marketing application for marketing thalidomide was reviewed by the F. D. A. for the United States in 1960 but was not approved because of concerns about peripheral neuropathy associated its use. While the agency was awaiting answers to these concerns, the link between thalidomide use and an epidemic of congenital malformations occurring in Europe exploded, an attributed to thalidomide in a letter, to the editor published by Lenz and McBride [7]. When taken in the first trimester of pregnancy, thalidomide prevented the proper growth of the fetus, resulting in nothing less than exceedingly rare, horrific birth defects and neonatal deaths. Any part of the fetus that was in development at the time of thalidomide ingestion could be affected. For those babies who survived, birth defects included deafness, blindness, disfigurement, cleft palate, many major internal disabilities, and the most common feature phecomelia (shortening of/ or the absence of limbs). Not only did a percentage of the population experience the effects of peripheral neuritis (numbness of the hands and feet) that was the F. D. A.'s original concern but thalidomide was revealed to be a catastrophic drug with tragic side effects The drug was withdrawn from the international market, and the tragedy played a part in the debate around the 1962 amendments to the Federal Food, Drug, and Cosmetic Act that resulted in specific effectiveness requirements for drugs.

The numbers vary from source to source, but it has been claimed that there were between ten thousand and twenty thousand babies born disabled as a consequence of the drug thalidomide. Two thirds of those victims born alive are now dead. An English report suggests that adult survivors of thalidomide exposure have a greater incidence of children with birth defects of the limbs [6]. The extremely low prevalence of the conditions (particularly phecomelia) in the general population compounded with the marked rise in prevalence after exposure, obviates the need for multiple studies replete with *p* values to infer causality.

The Radium Girls

"The doctors tell me I will die, but I mustn't. I have too much to live for—a husband who loves me and two children I adore. They say nothing can save me, nothing but a miracle." Ottawa native Catherine Donohue wrote those words and more from her bed to the Our Lady of Sorrows Roman Catholic Church in Chicago in the mid-1930s. She asked for a novena to bring her a miracle. She had to write the words, for she could not speak them. Her teeth and a large portion of her jawbone were gone. Cancer was eating away at her bone marrow. The doomed young mother weighed only 65 pounds [8]. Ms. Donohue was a charter member of "The Society of the Living Dead," so called because its members had two things in common: all worked at the Radium Dial Company in Ottawa, Illinois and all eventually suffered an agonizing death from radium radiation poison.

Luminescent numbers on wristwatches designed for soldiers involved in the trench warfare of World War I became a consumer fad in the 1920s. Attracted by easy work and high wages, young women, mostly young and unmarried, were employed to paint the dials of watches with self-illuminating paint containing the relatively new element radium.

Besides the promise of decent work for decent pay, Clark writes, part of what must have made dial painting an attractive job was working with such a sensational product; glow-in-the-dark paint. The young workers were excited about their jobs. They were told that they would be working with products that would "put a glow in [their] cheeks," Assured that the radium-laced compound was completely safe, even digestible, they painted their clothing, fingernails, and even their teeth, "for a smile that glowed in the dark." When they went home from work, they thrilled their families and friends with glowing clothes, fingers and hair.

Unfortunately, they were involved in lethal activity. Dial painters were instructed in the technique of "lip pointing" to perform their finely detailed work. Mixing the dry, luminous paint powder with paste and thinner, the workers drew their small brush to a point with their lips before dipping it in the paint, and then meticulously filled in the numbers or other marks on clock faces or other equipment before repeating the process. The greatest exposure to radium was in the mouth and jaws, and thirty women contracted bone cancer. Here again p values played no role in the assignment of causation. When the finding of exposure is specific enough and the disease is extremely rare causality is easily established with careful observation and deductive reasoning.

This is not to say that statistical inference should be avoided. However in some circumstances, the specificity of the disease, and the relationship between the occurrence of the disease and a new exposure, can call for a p value-less conclusion. Waiting for an additional study before one puts the final nail in the causality argument is sometimes a luxury which the medical community cannot afford. Such is the nature of the mathematics-ethics tension in medical research.

The Buy-In

In the two previous examples, p values were unnecessary to demonstrate a causal link. In other circumstances, the p value conveys important information. However, it is not all of the information.

Consider the findings of CARE [9]. This was a study to assess the benefits of cholesterol-reducing therapy in patients who have already sustained a heart attack and have normal cholesterol levels. The purpose of the study was to randomize approximately four thousand patients to either a cholesterol-reducing agent or a placebo, and follow them for five years. The clinical endpoint was fatal or nonfatal coronary artery disease. This experiment was considered ethical at the time, because no one knew whether patients who had had a previous heart attack, and with normal LDL cholesterol levels (115–175 mg/dl) would benefit from cholesterol-lowering therapy.

The results of CARE were phenomenal. In the active group, 10.2 percent of patients experienced a fatal or nonfatal heart attack, as compared to 13.2 percent of patients in the placebo group. The p value for this finding was very small, 0.003. Was this result clinically significant? The CARE investigators demonstrated that

---

[5] Described in chapter 10.

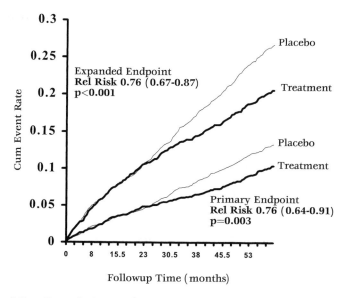

Figure 4.1. Cumulative Endpoint Event Rate by Therapy Group

this effect represented a 24 percent decrease in the risk of fatal and nonfatal coronary artery disease, and further revealed that if one thousand patients were treated for five years, thirty-seven coronary artery disease events (fatal or nonfatal heart attacks) would be prevented. If the one thousand patients were women, ninety-three events would be prevented. If the patients were greater than sixty years of age, seventy-three fatal or nonfatal coronary events would be prevented. These computations, when provided by the investigators provide additional context for the p value to be interpreted. However, there is yet an additional perspective to be considered.

Figure 4.1 demonstrates the effect of therapy for the primary endpoint (fatal and nonfatal myocardial infarction) and the expanded endpoint in CARE (primary endpoint plus revascularization). Note that the graph has a curious feature. For both the primary endpoint and the expanded endpoint, the experience of the placebo and treatment groups is identical for the first twenty-four months of follow-up. The beneficial effect of therapy appears only for patients who have been on therapy for two years. There is a payoff of therapy, but only after a two year buy-in or investment. The p value did not convey this important component of the information about the effect of therapy.

Do Blood Pressures Lie? The Frye Test

As lawsuits are commonly brought against pharmaceutical industries, and the dangers of breast implants, second hand smoke, and diet drugs are now having their days in court, the legal system is grappling with issues in epidemiology and biostatistics that used to be the exclusive domain of research scientists. It is useful to examine just how the legal system is coming to grips with significance testing and epidemiologic methods.

The first modern attempt to incorporate the role of science into the law was the Frye case. In the seventy years since its formulation, the "general acceptance" rule has been the dominant standard for determining the admissibility of scientific evidence at trial. Although under increasing attack of late, the rule continues to be followed by a majority of courts. In the Frye case, a court's decision was based on the reliability of a crude device that was a forerunner to the modern polygraph machine. This device measured systolic blood pressure, and surreptitiously attempted to gauge the veracity of a subject's statements by changes in that subject's blood pressure. In what has become a famous passage, the Court of Appeals of the District of Columbia described the device and its operation, declaring, "while courts will go a long way in admitting expert testimony deduced from a well-recognized scientific principle or discovery, the thing from which the deduction is made must be sufficiently established to have gained general acceptance in the particular field in which it belongs."[6] Because the systolic blood pressure deception test had not yet gained such standing and recognition among scientific authorities, evidence based on its results was ruled inadmissible. What was necessary was for the scientific community to have "generally accepted" the procedure.

The merits of the Frye test have been much debated. Opponents of the Frye test of general acceptability have focused on the establishment of federal Rules of Evidence. They believe that these rules superceded the Frye test. The Supreme Court agreed. Rule 402 of the Federal Rules of Evidence states that "All relevant evidence is admissible, except as otherwise provided by the Constitution of the United States, by Act of Congress, by these rules, or by other rules prescribed by the Supreme Court pursuant to statutory authority. Evidence which is not relevant is not admis-

[6] 54 App. D.C., at 47, 293 F., at 1014.

sible." Thus, after Frye, the test for evidence became one of relevance. The Court defined relevance as "any tendency to make the existence of any fact that is of consequence to the determination of the action more probable or less probable than it would be without the evidence." That is, if evidence adds to or subtracts from the plausibility of a useful fact in a case, the evidence is relevant. This idea, and liberal definition of relevancy of evidence, became the new standard of the Court, while the Court is also allowed to use the experience of common law.[7]

The Havner Ruling

Two critical cases have advanced and added important structure to the role of courts in establishing the legal interpretation of science in establishing or rebutting arguments in court. Both of these cases involve the drug Bendectin which was manufactured by Merrell Dow[8] and marketed since 1957. It was developed to fight morning sickness, and, before it was taken off the market, more than thirty-three million pregnant women took the drug.

The major health concern related to Bendectin was birth defects. It is notable and remarkable that, although Merrel-Dow was targeted by hundreds of Bendectin-injury lawsuits, each of these has ended in favor of the drug company (either at trial or on appeal). Two of those cases led to the establishment of rules for admissible scientific evidence. These rules are based on epidemiology and, to some degree involve p values.

After her mother was placed on a course of Bendectin in 1981, Kelly Havner was born with several missing fingers on her right hand. The Havners sued Merrell Dow for negligence, defective design, and defective marketing. The central issue in the case was the scientific reliability of the expert testimony offered to establish causation between the use of Bendectin and the occurrence of birth defects. Merrell Dow challenged the Havners' causation evidence, contending that there is no scientifically reliable evidence that Bendectin causes limb reduction birth defects or that it caused Kelly Havner's birth defect.

The basis of the arguments in the trial was the role of epidemiology in establishing the causative link. The Havners' experts

[7] In *United States* v. *Abel, 469 U.S. 45* (1984), the Supreme Court considered the pertinence of background common law in interpreting the Rules of Evidence.
[8] Now named Merrell Pharmaceuticals and a subsidiary of Hoechst Marion Roussel Inc.

were well credentialed. Shanna Helen Swan's testimony was central to their case. Dr. Swan, who held a master's degree in biostatistics from Columbia University and a doctorate in statistics from the University of California at Berkeley, was chief of the section of the California Department of Health and Services that determines causes of birth defects, and served as a consultant to the World Health Organization, the Food and Drug Administration, and the National Institutes of Health. Dr. Stewart A. Newman was a professor at New York Medical College and had spent over a decade studying the effect of chemicals on limb development. After exhaustive analyses, these experts had concluded that Bendectin could cause birth defects. Their conclusions were based upon; in vitro and in vivo animal studies that found a link between Bendectin and malformations; pharmacological studies of the chemical structure of Bendectin that purported to show similarities between the structure of the drug and that of other substances known to cause birth defects; and the "reanalysis" of previously published epidemiological studies.

The question of scientific reliability was raised repeatedly during the liability phase, at the center of which was the role of epidemiology and animal studies. At the conclusion of the liability phase, the jury found in favor of the Havners and awarded them $3.75 million. In the punitive damages stage, the jury awarded another $30 million, but that amount was reduced by the trial court to $15 million. However, the manufacturer appealed, and a Texas state appeals court threw out the punitive-damages award and ruled that the Havners were entitled to only the $3.75 million in compensatory damages. Later the Texas Supreme Court ruled that Havner was not entitled to any award at all because there had been insufficient evidence linking Bendectin to birth defects. In doing so, it sifted through how weight should be apportioned to scientific evidence.

The issue before the Supreme Court, as in most of the Bendectin cases, was whether the Havners' evidence was scientifically reliable. The Havners did not contend that all limb reduction birth defects were caused by Bendectin or that Bendectin always caused limb reduction birth defects, even when taken at the critical time of limb development. Experts for the Havners and Merrell Dow agreed that some limb reduction defects are genetic. These experts also agreed that the cause of a large percentage of limb reduction birth defects is unknown. Given these undisputed facts, the court wrestled with just what a plaintiff must establish to raise the issue of whether Bendectin caused an individual's birth defect (i.e., specific causation).

The Havners relied to a considerable extent on epidemiological studies for proof of general causation. Accordingly, the Supreme Court considered and accepted the use of epidemiological studies and the "more likely than not" burden of proof. The Supreme Court recognized, as does the federal *Reference Manual on Scientific Evidence,* that unfocused data such as the incidence of adverse effects in the exposed population cannot indicate the actual cause of a given individual's disease or condition. The Court noted that sound methodology requires that the design and execution of epidemiological studies be examined, especially to control the factor of bias[9]. The Court stated that epidemiological studies "are subject to many biases and therefore present formidable problems in design and execution and even greater problems in interpretation."[10,11]

The Supreme Court identified several reasons why the plaintiffs' expert opinions were scientifically unreliable. First, Dr. Swan provided an odds ratio of 2.8 with no confidence interval. The Court stated that, without knowing the significance level or the confidence interval, there was no scientifically reliable basis for saying that the 2.8 result is an indication of anything. Further, the court noted that the expert's choice of the control group could have skewed the results (Dr. Swan testified at trial that she chose births of Down's Syndrome babies).

In addition to the statistical shortcomings of the Havners' epidemiological evidence, the Court criticized the evidence's reliability because it had never been published or otherwise subjected to peer review, with the exception of Dr. Swan's abstract, which she acknowledged was not the equivalent of a published paper. None of the findings offered by the Havners' five experts in this case have been published, studied, or replicated by the relevant scientific community. As Judge Kozinski said, "The only review the plaintiffs' experts' work has received has been by judges and juries, and the only place their theories and studies have been published is in the pages of federal and state reporters."[11] The

---

[9] Discussed in Chapter 3.

[10] *Daubert,* 43 F.3d at 1318 (commenting on the same five witnesses called by the Havners).

[11] The controversy on the role of epidemiology continues to rage, most recently in diet drug litigation.

Supreme Court identified several factors to consider, including whether the study was prepared only for litigation or used or relied upon outside the courtroom; whether the methodology was recognized in the scientific community; and has the litigation spawned its own "community" that is not part of the purely scientific community. The Court observed that the opinions to which the Havners' witnesses testified had never been offered outside the confines of a courthouse. In doing so, the Court recognized that publication and peer review allow an opportunity for the relevant scientific community to comment on findings and conclusions and to replicate the reported results using different populations and different study designs.

Relative Risk and the Supreme Court

Although they discounted the specific evidence offered in Havner, the Supreme Court stated that properly designed and executed epidemiological studies may be part of the evidence supporting causation in such a case. The Court went even further, setting a legal standard for strength of evidence, by stating that there was a rational basis for the requirement that there be more than a "doubling of the risk." Thus the court required a relative risk, or odds ratio, of two.[12] However, the Court cautioned that other factors must be considered because a relative risk of more than 2.0 is not a litmus test. The use of scientifically reliable epidemiological studies and the requirement of more than a doubling of the risk strikes a balance between the needs of our legal system and the limits of science. The Court recognized that few courts have embraced the more-than-double-the-risk standard and indicated that in some instances, epidemiological studies with relative risks of less than 2.0 might suffice if there were other evidence of causation. However, it was unwilling to decide in this case whether epidemiological evidence with a relative risk less than 2.0, coupled with other credible and reliable evidence, may be legally sufficient to support causation.[13] The Court did empha-

---

[12] A relative risk of two is equivalent to an attributable risk exposed of 0.50.

[13] For example, see *Daubert,* 43 F.3d at 1321 n.16; *Hall,* 947 F.Supp. at 1398, 1404.

size, that evidence of causation from any source must have its scientific reliability considered, and it would not admit post hoc speculative testimony. For example, the court noted that a treating physician or other expert who has seen a skewed data sample, such as one of a few infants who have a birth defect, is not in a position to infer causation.[14] The scientific community should not accept as methodologically sound a "study" by such an expert, reporting that the ingestion of a particular drug by the mother caused the birth defect. Similarly, an expert's assertion that a physical examination confirmed causation should not be accepted at face value. Further, the court cautioned that an expert cannot dissect a study, picking and choosing data, or "reanalyze" the data to derive a higher relative risk if this process does not comport with sound scientific methodology.

P Values, Confidence Intervals and the Courts

The Court stated that it is unwise to depart from the methodology that is at present generally accepted among epidemiologists, writing that allmost all thoughtful scientists would agree that a significance level of five percent is a reasonable general standard.[15] The Court resisted attempts to widen the boundaries at which courts will acknowledge a statistically significant association beyond the 95 percent level. Thus the court seems to accept the notion of significance testing and the Fisher 0.05 standard for significance testing. In addition, the Court recognized that the establishment of an association does not indicate causality. It stated that even if a statistically significant association is found, that association does not equate to causation. As the original panel of the court of appeals observed in this case, there is a demonstrable association between summertime and death by drowning, but summertime does not cause drowning.

---

[14] The reasons for this are discussed in Chapter 1, "Patients, patience, and p values".

[15] A fine discussion of this concept appears in the Amicus Curiae Brief of Professor Alvan R. Feinstein in Support of Respondent at 16, *Daubert v. Merrell Dow Pharms., Inc.*, 509 U.S. 579, 113 S.Ct. 2786, 125 L.Ed.2d 469 (1993) (No. 92–102).

In the final analysis, the Court held there was no scientifically reliable evidence to support the judgment in the Havners' case. Accordingly, it reversed part of the judgment of the lower court and rendered judgment for Merrell Dow. However, the Havner case firmly established the importance of epidemiology, peer reviewed published results, and, through a statement about confidence intervals, the role of statistical inference in making legal arguments for causation.

The Daubert Rulings

The Daubert case, also involving Bendectin, allowed the legal system to elaborate on the question of who should assess the validity of the evidence for causality. Jason Daubert and Eric Schuller were children born with serious birth defects. They and their parents sued Merrell Dow in California state court, alleging that the birth defects had been caused by the mothers' ingestion of Bendectin. Merrell Dow had the suits moved to federal court. After extensive examination of all the facts by both the plaintiffs' and defendant's attorneys, the drug company moved for summary judgment (i.e., for the case to be thrown out), contending that Bendectin does not cause birth defects in humans and that the Dauberts' would be unable to come forward with any admissible evidence that it does. In support of its motion, the drug company submitted an affidavit from Steven H. Lamm, physician and epidemiologist, who was a well-credentialed expert on the risks from exposure to various chemical substances. Doctor Lamm stated that he had reviewed all the literature on Bendectin and human birth defects — more than thirty published studies involving over 130,000 patients. In his view, no study had found Bendectin to be a human teratogen (i.e.,, a substance capable of causing malformations in fetuses). On the basis of this review, Doctor Lamm concluded that maternal use of Bendectin during the first trimester of pregnancy had not been shown to be a risk factor for human birth defects.

The Dauberts did not contest this characterization of the published record regarding Bendectin. Instead, they responded to the manufacturer's motion with the testimony of eight experts of their own, each of whom also possessed impressive credentials. The Dauberts also responded with both animal data and epidemiological studies and analyses. However, the District Court granted Merrell Dow's motion for summary judgment. Given the vast body of epidemiological data concerning Bendectin, the court held, expert opinion that is not based on epidemiological evidence is not admissible to establish causation. Thus, the animal cell studies, live animal studies, and chemical structure analyses on which the Dauberts had relied could not by themselves raise a reasonably disputable jury issue regarding causation. Furthermore, the Dauberts' epidemiological analyses, based as they were on recalculations of data in previously published studies that had found no causal link between the drug and birth defects, were ruled to be inadmissible because they had not been published or subjected to peer review. When the Daubert case went to the United States Supreme Court, the Court let stand the lower court rulings in favor of Merrell Dow. The justices also stated that, faced with the possibility of expert scientific testimony, the trial judge must determine at the outset whether the expert is proposing to provide scientific knowledge that will assist the court to understand or determine the important issues. The Court said that this examination would entail a preliminary assessment of whether the reasoning or methodology underlying the testimony was scientifically valid and of whether that reasoning or methodology could properly be applied to the facts at issue.

The trial judge must make this preliminary assessment in what are now known as Daubert hearings. This inquiry will include many considerations; whether the theory or technique in question can be (and has been) tested, whether it has been subjected to peer review and publication; its known or potential error rate; the existence and maintenance of standards controlling its operation; and whether it has attracted widespread acceptance within a relevant scientific community. The inquiry is a flexible one, and its focus must be solely on principles and methodology, not on the conclusions that they generate. The Supreme Court ruled that judges (at least federal judges) were competent to undertake this review, and then proceeded to provide some guidance for them.

First, the scientific statement must be capable of being tested. "Scientific methodology today is based on generating hypotheses and testing them to see if they can be falsified; indeed, this methodology is what distinguishes science from other fields of human inquiry. The methodology used by the experts must itself have been put to the scrutiny of other scientist. Another pertinent consideration was whether the theory or technique has been exposed to peer review and publication. Publication is but one element of peer review and not a requirement of admissibility does not necessarily correlate with reliability and in some instances well grounded but innovative theories will not have been published. Submission to the scrutiny of the scientific community is a component of "good science," in part because it increases the likelihood that substantive flaws in methodology will be detected. The fact of publication (or lack thereof) in a peer reviewed journal will thus be a relevant consideration in assessing the scientific validity of a particular technique or methodology on which an opinion is premised. Additionally, in the case of a particular scientific technique, the court should consider the known or potential rate of error[16] and the existence and maintenance of standards controlling the technique's operation.[17] Finally, "general acceptance", the standard set in *Frye,* may yet have a bearing on the inquiry in the preliminary hearing.

The opinion of the Court was that this preliminary hearing on the admissibility of the scientific evidence, in combination with vigorous cross-examination, presentation of contrary evidence, and careful instruction on the burden of proof is the traditional and appropriate means of assessing shaky but admissible evidence.

Conclusions

P values may be desirable, but they are sometimes unnecessary, as experience with the radium girls and thalidomide has demonstrated. Sometimes *p* values do not convey the relative unimportance of an effect size. Sometimes they do not convey the way in which the effect size is received. The final indicator of the value of a beneficial interaction is not the *p* value, but the benefit. If a substance is associated with a harmful effect, focus finally on the effect and its implications, not just on its *p* value.

The courts admit that they lag behind science in determining the scientific merit of a legal argument. However, in the past twenty years they have come to rely on the findings of epidemiology and biostatistics to buttress or rebut an argument. However, the court has allowed judges to see for themselves the merits of the scientific argument before a jury hears it. Many of the rules

[16] *United States* v. *Smith,*869 F. 2d 348, 353–354 is an interesting case involving the survey of error rates in spectrographic voice identification technique.
[17] See *United States* v. *Williams,* 583 F. 2d 1194, 1198 (CA2 1978).

established by the Supreme Court to guide judges in these preliminary hearings are based on the criteria in this book, e.g. reproducibility, timing, significance of the association.

References

1. Noremberg, D., LRC, (1996) Letter to the Editor. *JAMA* 252:2545.
2. Abenhaim, L., Moride, Y., and Brenot, F., (1996) "Appetite-suppressant drugs and the risk of primary pulmonary hypertension," International Pulmonary Hypertension Study Groups [see comments], *N Engl J Med* 335:609–616.
3. Ouellet, B.L., Romeder, J.M. and Lance, J.M., (1979b) "Premature mortality attributable to smoking and hazardous drinking in Canada," *Am. J. Epidemiology* 109:451–463.
4. Thompson, W.D., (1987) "Statistical criteria in the interpretation of epidemiologic data (Different views)," *American Journal of Public Health* 77:191–194.
5. Poole, C., (1987) "Beyond the confidence interval," *American Journal of Public Health* 77:195–199.
6. Times Newspaper Ltd., The Sunday Times of London, (1979) "Suffer the Children: The Story of Thalidomide.
7. Lenz, W., (1962) "Thalidomide and Congenital Abnormalities," (Letter to the Editor) *Lancet* 1:45.
8. Clark, C., (1997) *Radium Girls: Women and Industrial Health Reform, 1910–1935*, University of North Carolina Press, Chapel Hill, NC.
9. Sacks, F.M., Pfeffer, M.A., and Moye, L.A., Rouleau, J.L., Rutherford, J.D., Cole, T.G., Brown, L., Warnica, J.W., Arnold, J.M.O., Wun, C.C., Davis, B.R., Braunwald, E. for the Cholesterol and recurrent Events Trial Investigators, (1996) "The effect of pravastatin on coronary events after myocardial infarction in patients with average cholesterol levels," *N Engl J Med* 335:1001–1009.

5

CHAPTER

"Your Searchlight's Not On!" Power and *P* Values

Consider an experiment which is coming to an end. At its conclusion, the experiment's prinicple investigator often feels hemmed in, cornered, and eventually trapped by persistent critics. They left him alone during both the design and the execution of the experiment. However, as soon as he attempts to draw a conclusion from his sample, hesitant and circumspect as these conclusions may be, the specter of sampling error rises up. Even if the results are negative, demonstrating no relationship between the treatment and the disease, the critics close in, asking now about type II error. Isn't it possible that there was an effect in the population, but, again through the play of chance, the population produced for the investigator a sample that demonstrated no relationship. Critics relentlessly remind him that his findings may be nothing at all, merely the vicissitude of the population., Like a weed, sampling error rises up to strangle the early blossom of his result. Is there no hope?

The answer is power! By its very nature it sounds like something we can't do without. *P* values seem complicated, slithery, and mysterious. Power speaks with purpose, focus and direction. Convince us with *p* values, if you must, but give us power! There is hope here, and just a little trouble as well.

120

The Critic's View

Research program critics generally and appropriately want to know one thing: How likely is it that the investigator has been misled? The content of the research investigator's conclusion— positve or negativee—does not matter. Colleagues and critics want to know the likelihood that the conclusion is wrong. Consider an experiment in which an investigator wishes to demonstrate that her treatment for ischemic heart disease will produce a 20 percent reduction in the risk of fatal and nonfatal myocardial infarction. She correctly anticipates that her critics will want to know how likely it is that she is being misled by her sample. If she executed her significance test from a concordantly executed experiment concluding that the treatment effect is present, her critics will ask. How likely is it that this treatment effect, so apparent in your sample, is not present in the population? How likely is it that, in the population, the treatment produces no efficacy, but you have been fooled by a sample in which efficacy appeared to be present? We recognize this question as an issue involving type I sampling error and is addressed by an *a priori* allocation of alpha and by the p value at the trial's conclusion. If the experiment is concordantly executed, the p value is interpretable.

However, there is another sampling error issue. What is the correct conclusion of the experiment if the investigator's test statistic did not fall into the critical region? Does this finding imply that the treatment is not successful and will not produce the required level of efficacy in the population? This is also a conclusion with important implications, and again the critics home in, armed with a different question. How likely is it that the treatment is effective in the population, but the population has misled the investigator by producing a sample that shows no efficacy? This is the type II error.

Let's consider the thought process of this error in more detail. The investigator's significance test falls in the critical region and critics wonder about the spectrum of samples produced from a population in which there is no efficacy. The population produces many samples, some of which will mirror efficacy and some of which will not. In this circumstance, the issue is one of minimizing the probability that the population will produce a sample that appears to suggest efficacy. However, for the type II error, we shift the paradigm, assuming not as before that there was no efficacy in the population, but instead, assuming that there is efficacy of the treatment in the population. If this treatment effect is present in the population, we wish the sample to reflect it. The probability that the sample does not reflect this positive population finding is termed the *probability of type II error*, or the *beta error*.

It has become common for investigators to refer to the beta error subtracted from one. This new quantity is called the *power* of the experiment. The power of an experiment is the probability that the population in which the treatment is effective produces a sample that mirrors this effect, i.e. that a population with embedded efficacy produces a sample with embedded efficacy. Unlike alpha, power is to be maximized. The greater the power, the more confidence we have that the population has not misled us.

We all like power. However sometimes we are unwilling to pay the sample size price to retain it. Power is crucial in experimental interpretation. Experiments in which the null hypothesis is rejected are called *positive*. However, what is the correct conclusion if the null hypothesis is not rejected? Can we term such results negative? Only when there is adequate power. Power is critical in experimental interpretation, especially and primarily if the *p* value is large. In this circumstance, there is sometimes irrisitable temptation to call the experiment negative, and to call the treatments equivalent. However, the lower power level tells us that it is quite possible that the population contains treatment difference, but produced a sample suggesting no benefit of therapy. Therefore, since the probability of being misled by a nonrepresentative sample is high, equivalence in the sample does not translate to treatment equivalence in the population. With adequate power, the likelihood of a misleading sample is small, and we are confident in translating sample treatment equivalence to population treatment equivalence.

Suppose I tell a friend of mine, "I know that in the basement of this house there is a precious jewel. Go down, find it, and make us both rich." My friend immediately begins the search, but after many minutes, returns, tired and soiled, replying quietly, "My friend, the jewel is not there—but I never turned the light on". Can I believe the jewel is missing? How can I believe the conclusion of the search if the search was flawed? Even if the jewel was there, he would not have found it, so how can I believe there is no jewel just because he says there is none? An underpowered research effort is a search with the lights turned off. We will very likely never find the jewel. For our (re)search to be persuasive, we must have our searchlights on.

No Way Out?

We know that the smaller the alpha error, the better. Now we know that the greater the power, the better. However, we cannot, (touching no other part of the experiment), decrease alpha without decreasing power, nor can we increase power without increasing the type I error. The thought process is very revealing here. Suppose we want to change the experiment by decreasing the alpha error. By reducing the alpha error, we reduce the probability that the population with equivalent treatments will produce samples with treatment efficacy. How do we specifically decrease this probability? We do this by making the criteria for efficacy in the sample very strong, "extremely extreme." However, if we make the criteria extreme, it is possible that moderate efficacy will be embedded in the sample but, because it does not meet the extreme criteria,will not appear in the sample and will be interpreted as no effect. Thus, if there was efficacy in the population, it is possible that this efficacy signal would not be transmitted to the sample since the new criteria were so extreme. Our attempt to reduce the likelihood of an alpha error has made it easier for us to miss efficacy in our sample, if there is in fact efficacy in the population. We have overtly diminished alpha but inadvertently diminished power as well.

However, there is a way out. The only way to simultaneously minimize alpha and maximize power is to increase the number of observations. By increasing the size of the sample, the investigator improves the precision of the efficacy estimate, making it easier to distinquish between the distribution of the efficacy measure under the null hypothesis from its distribution under the alternative hypothesis. Thus, sample size computations are critical in insuring that the investigator has the correct balance of alpha and power.

Sample Size Computations

The most important lesson to learn about sample size computations is that they are often not about sample size at all. The computations may have been initially motivated by stark concerns about alpha and power but they serve as a strong political gravity well, attracting the important trial forces with their differing goals. Thus the computations act as a strong political gravity well, bringing people with a stake in the trial together to discuss and settle on the trial's purpose. Sample size computations are the table over which important trial agendas meet and collide, ultimately deciding the purpose and direction of the experiment.

This is not sinister; in fact, it is very appropriate and, when the conversations are frank and meaningful, gives the experiment a much better chance for success. During this period of the design of the experiment, there are several corps of workers. There are the investigators, who possess clinical insight about the experiment, are knowledgeable about the clinical condition, and, have experience with the intervention. There is also a corps of epidemiologists and biostatisticians, who have the capability of assessing strengths and weaknesses of experimental designs, and who identify the frequency with which the endpoint of the trial will occur. Finally, there are also the administrators, who will be involved in planning the logistics of and paying for the experiment. Early in the trial's design phase, discussions proceed largely within each of these groups, investigators discussing patient selection issues and clinical efficacy, epidemiologists and biostatisticians discussing event rates, and statistical efficacy and administrators discussing costs and funding. It is the sample size computation that brings these corps into direct contact. Each group contributes a critical assumption or data to the discussion, and, in the process reveals its own thought processes as the other corps reveal theirs. It is frank, refreshing and, when collegially handled, results in a strong trial design. The resulting sample size is mathematically consistent and logical, to be sure, but also integrates the necessary logistical and financial considerations. The sample size computation is the anvil on which the trial design is finally hammered.

To the uninitiated, sample size computations seem like an impenetrable maze of mysterious calculations and slippery probability statements. They are actually very straightforward, with many sources in the literature [1–5 as examples]. We will provide a heavily guided demonstration of the formulas involved in two common scenarios. The first scenario will compute the sample size for and experiment with a continuous outcome—left ventricular end diastolic volume. The second scenario will work through the computation for the discrete (statisticians sometimes call this dichotomous) outcome of total mortality. For each demonstration, there will be three phases of the computation.

Phase I—under the null
Phase II—under the alternative
Phase III—consolidation

Continuous Outcome Measures

Consider a randomized controlled clinical trial designed to test the effect of an intervention on the change in left ventricular end diastolic volume (EDV). Patients are recruited using a random sampling plan and have their baseline EDV measured. They are then randomized to receive placebo care or the intervention, and followed for three months, at the end of which they have their EDV measured again. The investigator assumes that the EDVs will be normally distributed, and wishes to analyze the change in EDV over time across the two groups. He believes that there will be a large increase in EDV in the placebo group, reflecting the natural progression of the disease. It is his hope that the EDV change will be smaller in the treatment arm of the experiment.

To simplify some, let $\mu(d_x)$ be the population mean change in the end diastolic volumes for the placebo group and $\mu(d_y)$ be the population mean change in the end diastolic volume in the active group. Let's begin with the null hypothesis

$$H_0 : \mu(d_x) = \mu(d_y) \text{ vs. } H_a : \mu(d_x) \,|\, \mu(d_y)$$

Clearly, the investigator does not believe the alternative hypothesis as stated, he believes that $\mu(d_x)$ the population mean change in EDV in the placebo group, will be greater than $\mu(d_y)$, the population mean change in EDV in the active group. However, since he recognizes that he does not know the effect of therapy, he states the alternative hypothesis as two sided[1]. However, his true belief in the ability of the treatment to affect the change in EDV will be reflected in phase II.

Phase I—The null hypothesis
The purpose of phase I is simply to construct the test statistic and identify its critical region. The distribution of the test statistic is the distribution under the null hypothesis, i.e. under the assumption that there is no treatment effect on the mean change in EDV. As was stated before, the investigator believes the difference in

---

[1] This notion of test sidedness is discussed in Chapter 5.

EDVs will follow a normal distribution. Let d_x be the sample mean change in the placebo group, and d_y is the sample mean change in the active group. Let $Var[d_x - d_y]$ be the variance of the difference in chance of the EDVs We note that under the null hypothesis the quantity

$$\frac{d_x - d_y}{\sqrt{Var[d_x - d_y]}} \tag{5.1}$$

follows a normal distribution. Then the null hypothesis will be rejected when

$$\frac{d_x - d_y}{\sqrt{Var[d_x - d_y]}} > Z_{1-\alpha/2} \tag{5.2}$$

where $Z_{1-\alpha/2}$ is the $1 - \alpha/2$ percentile value from the standard normal distribution mean zero and variance one. We may rewrite equation 5.2 to see that we will reject the null hypothesis in favor of the alternate

$$d_x - d_y > Z_{1-\alpha/2}\sqrt{Var[d_x - d_y]} \tag{5.3}$$

This ends phase I.

Phase II — The alternative hypothesis
This next phase incorporates the result of phase I with the notion of power.

Begin with the definition of power

Power = Prob[The null hypothesis is rejected | the alternative hypothesis is true]

The null hypothesis is rejected when the test statistic falls in the critical region. The alternative hypothesis is true if $\mu(d_x) - \mu(d_y) = \Delta > 0$. This quantity Δ is the difference that the investigator hopes to see between the changes in the two groups. This consideration is not two sided at this point, and is the opportunity for the investigator to state precisely state the magnitude of efficacy he believes this treatment will produce.

Using the result of Phase I we can write the power equation as

$$Power = P[d_x - d_y > Z_{1-\alpha/2}\sqrt{Var[d_x - d_y]} \,|\, \Delta] \tag{5.4}$$

We now standardize this so that the quantity on the left follows a standard normal distribution. Under phase II, the alternative hypothesis the mean of $\mu(d_x) - \mu(d_y) = \Delta > 0$. This leads to

$$Power = P\left[\frac{d_x - d_y - \Delta}{\sqrt{Var[d_x - d_y]}} > \frac{Z_{1-\alpha/2}\sqrt{Var[d_x - d_y]} - \Delta}{\sqrt{Var[d_x - d_y]}}\right] \quad (5.5)$$

$$= P\left[\frac{d_x - d_y - \Delta}{\sqrt{Var[d_x - d_y]}} > Z_{1-\alpha/2} - \frac{\Delta}{\sqrt{Var[d_x - d_y]}}\right] \quad (5.6)$$

$$= P\left[N(0,1) > Z_{1-\alpha/2} - \frac{\Delta}{\sqrt{Var[d_x - d_y]}}\right] \quad (5.7)$$

These steps are simply algebra. From the last step we know Prob $[N(0,1) > Z_\beta] = 1 - \beta$, so we can now write

$$Z_\beta = Z_{1-\alpha/2} - \frac{\Delta}{\sqrt{Var[d_x - d_y]}} \quad (5.8)$$

This concludes Phase II.

Phase III Consolidation

Phase III concluded with an equation, which we must now solve for n. The sample size n is embedded in the variance term in the denominator of equation 5.8.

$$Var[d_x - d_y] = \frac{\sigma_D^2}{n} + \frac{\sigma_D^2}{n} = \frac{2\sigma_D^2}{n} \quad (5.9)$$

Where σ_D^2 is the variance of an intrasubject difference. Note that the n in the equation represents the group size (placebo group or treatment group). The trial size N (i.e. the total number of subjects needed for the experiment) $= 2n$. The equation at the end of phase II can be rewritten as

$$Z_\beta = Z_{1-\alpha/2} - \frac{\Delta}{\sqrt{\frac{2\sigma_D^2}{n}}} \quad (5.10)$$

We need only solve this equation for n:

$$n = \frac{2\sigma_D^2[Z_{1-\alpha/2} - Z_\beta]^2}{\Delta^2} \quad (5.11)$$

and the trial size, N is

$$N = \frac{4\sigma_D^2[Z_{1-\alpha/2} - Z_\beta]^2}{\Delta^2} \quad (5.12)$$

To compute the power one need only adapt the following equation from Phase II

$$1 - \beta = P\left[N(0,1) > Z_{1-\alpha/2} - \frac{\Delta}{\sqrt{Var[d_x - d_y]}}\right] \qquad (5.13)$$

and rewrite the variance to find

$$1 - \beta = P\left[N(0,1) > Z_{1-\alpha/2} - \frac{\Delta}{\sqrt{\frac{2\sigma_D^2}{n}}}\right] \qquad (5.14)$$

Example:
If, for this experiment, the investigator chooses a two-sided alpha of 0.05, 90 percent power (beta = 0.10), delta = 10 and σ = 18, the trial size is

$$N = \frac{4\sigma^2[Z_{1-\alpha/2} - Z_\beta]^2}{[\Delta]^2} = \frac{4(18)^2[1.96 - (-1.28)]^2}{[10]^2} = 136 \qquad (5.15)$$

Or 68 subjects per group. If the delta of interest is 5 rather than 10, the power is

$$1 - \beta = P\left[N(0,1) > Z_{1-\alpha/2} - \frac{\Delta}{\sqrt{\frac{2\sigma^2}{n}}}\right]$$

$$= P\left[N(0,1) > 1.96 - \frac{5}{\sqrt{\frac{2(18)^2}{68}}}\right]$$

$$= P[N(0,1) > 0.34] = 0.37 \qquad (5.16)$$

Dichotamous Outcome Measures

The following example outlines the sample size for dichotomous outcome. Consider an experiment where the investigator wishes to demonstrate that her intervention will produce an important reduction in total mortality. The investigator recruits her patients, and randomly assigns them to the placebo group or to the intervention group. She will follow all of her patients for three years, counting the number of deaths. We will proceed as we did above, working through each of the three phases. As before, we start with the null hypothesis

$$H_0 : \rho_x = \rho_y, \text{ vs. } H_a : \rho_x \neq \rho_y.$$

Phase I — The null hypothesis.

As before, we take the opportunity to construct the test statistic. Let p_x be the sample estimate of total mortality rate for the placebo group, and p_y be the sample estimate of the total mortality rate of the treatment group. We note that under the null hypothesis the quantity

$$\frac{p_x - p_y}{\sqrt{Var[p_x - p_y]}} \tag{5.17}$$

follows a normal distribution with mean zero and variance one. Then, the null hypothesis will be rejected when

$$\frac{p_x - p_y}{\sqrt{Var[p_x - p_y]}} > Z_{1-\alpha/2} \tag{5.18}$$

or

$$p_x - p_y > Z_{1-\alpha/2}\sqrt{Var[p_x - p_y]}. \tag{5.19}$$

This ends phase I.

Phase II — The alternative hypothesis

As before, we begin with the definition of power

power = Prob [the null hypothesis is rejected |
the alternative hypothesis is true]

The null hypothesis is rejected when the test statistic falls in the critical region. The alternative hypothesis is true if $p_x - p_y = \Delta \neq 0$.

Using the result of Phase I we can write the power equation as

$$Power = P[p_x - p_y > Z_{1-\alpha/2}\sqrt{Var[p_x - p_y]} \,|\, \Delta] \tag{5.20}$$

We now standardize the argument in the probability statement of equation 5.20 so that the quantity on the left follows a standard normal distribution. This requires subtracting the population mean effect under the alternative distribution) and dividing by the square root of the variance of $p_x - p_y$. This process proceeds.

$$Power = P\left[\frac{p_x - p_y - \Delta}{\sqrt{Var[p_x - p_y]}} > \frac{Z_{1-\alpha/2}\sqrt{Var[p_x - p_y]} - \Delta}{\sqrt{Var[p_x - p_y]}}\right] \qquad (5.21)$$

$$= P\left[\frac{p_x - p_y - \Delta}{\sqrt{Var[p_x - p_y]}} > Z_{1-\alpha/2} - \frac{\Delta}{\sqrt{Var[p_x - p_y]}}\right] \qquad (5.22)$$

$$= P\left[N(0,1) > Z_{1-\alpha/2} - \frac{\Delta}{\sqrt{Var[p_x - p_y]}}\right] \qquad (5.23)$$

but of course this quantity is the power $= 1 - \beta$. By the definition of a percentile value we can now write

$$Z_\beta = Z_{1-\alpha/2} - \frac{\Delta}{\sqrt{Var[p_x - p_y]}}. \qquad (5.24)$$

Phase III–Consolidation.
Phase II concluded with an equation, which we must now solve for n. The sample size n is embedded in the variance term in the denominator.

$$Var[p_x - p_y] = \frac{p_x(1 - p_x)}{n} + \frac{p_y(1 - p_y)}{n} \qquad (5.25)$$

Note that the n in the equation is that for the group size. The trial size (i.e., the total number of subjects needed for the experiment) $N = 2n$. The equation at the end of phase II can be rewritten as

$$Z_\beta = Z_{1-\alpha/2} - \frac{\Delta}{\sqrt{Var[p_x - p_y]}} = Z_{1-\alpha/2} - \frac{\Delta}{\sqrt{\frac{p_x(1 - p_x)}{n} + \frac{p_y(1 - p_y)}{n}}}. \qquad (5.26)$$

We only need solve this equation for n:

$$n = \frac{[p_x(1 - p_x) + p_y(1 - p_y)][Z_{1-\alpha/2} - Z_\beta]^2}{\Delta^2}. \qquad (5.27)$$

and the trial size N is

$$N = \frac{2[p_x(1 - p_x) + p_y(1 - p_y)][Z_{1-\alpha/2} - Z_\beta]^2}{\Delta^2} \qquad (5.28)$$

To compute the power one need only adapt the following equation from Phase II

$$1 - \beta = P\left[N(0,1) > Z_{1-\alpha/2} - \frac{\Delta}{\sqrt{Var[p_x - p_y]}}\right] \qquad (5.29)$$

and rewrite the variance to find

$$1 - \beta = P\left[N(0,1) > Z_{1-\alpha/2} - \frac{\Delta}{\sqrt{Var[p_x - p_y]}}\right]$$

$$= P\left[N(0,1) > Z_{1-\alpha/2} - \frac{\Delta}{\sqrt{\dfrac{p_x(1 - p_x)}{n} + \dfrac{p_y(1 - p_y)}{n}}}\right]$$

Example:

If the experiment is designed for a two sided alpha of 0.05, 90 percent power (beta = 0.10), $p_1 = 0.20$, and efficacy = .25 (i.e., $p_2 = (0.20)(0.75) = 0.15$. Then $\Delta = 0.20 - 0.15$, the trial size is

$$N = \frac{2[p_x(1 - p_x) + p_y(1 - p_y)][Z_{1-\alpha/2} - Z_\beta]^2}{[p_x - p_y]^2}$$

$$= \frac{2[(0.20)(0.80) + (0.15)(0.85)][1.96 - (-1.28)]^2}{[0.20 - 0.15]^2} = 2414 \qquad (5.31)$$

or 1207 subjects per group. If only 1000 subjects per group can be identified the power is

$$Power = P\left[N(0,1) > Z_{1-\alpha/2} - \frac{\Delta}{\sqrt{\dfrac{p_x(1 - p_x)}{n} + \dfrac{p_y(1 - p_y)}{n}}}\right] \qquad (5.32)$$

$$= P\left[N(0,1) > 1.96 - \frac{0.05}{\sqrt{\dfrac{(0.20)(0.80)}{1000} + \dfrac{(0.15)(0.85)}{1000}}}\right] = 0.84$$

From these computations, we see that the sample size is a function of the expected effect size, the type I error and the type II error. It is also a function of the natural history of the disease process. However, we also know that we must introduce other considerations into this "political arithmetic"[2]

---

[2] See prologue.

The Right Sample Size —
Lipid Research Clinics

The sample size formulas designed above explicitly include important statistical concepts. However, these same formula also specifically exclude considerations that must be factored in to a sample size consideration. Chief among these are costs, both in resources and in finances. The above calculations serve no good purpose if they are followed blindly. The calculation may dictate that fourteen thousand patients should be randomized when only seven thousand patients are available. The cost of the trial size as computed may be $30,000,000, when only $3,000,000 is available. These considerations of resource availability are important, if not paramount, yet they are not explicitly considered in the sample size design. This is because they are folded in to the estimates for event rates and efficacy.

This is not to say that the event rates are rendered imprecise because of logistical considerations. Quite to the contrary, the event rates estimates are clearly sheathed in epidemiology and biostatistics. However, cost and other factors, which show up in the sample size computations, influence the design, direction and goal of the trial. The Lipid Research Clinics (LRC) trial was an important experiment examining the role of cholesterol management and reductions in morbidity and mortality in atherosclerotic cardiovascular disease. The difficulties and compromises achieved during its sample size computation serves as a good example of meshing logistical concerns with sample size computations.

As originally conceived, LRC would test the ability of a cholesterol reducing agent, cholestyramine, to reduce the number of mortal events. Men between thirty-five and sixty years of age with total cholesterol levels greater than 265 mg/dl would be randomized to receive either diet alone or diet plus cholestyramine for the management of their lipid levels. Patients would be followed for seven years. The endpoint of the study was coronary heart disease death, essentially fatal myocardial infarction. The sample size estimate returned by the statisticians was, depending upon the assumptions for type I/type II error rates, between twelve thousand and fifteen thousand patients. However, the investigators believed that they could only randomize and follow between three thousand and five thousand patients. The sample size required was 3–4 times beyond their ability to recruit patients.

It is important to first note what the investigators correctly chose not to do. They did not sanction the sample size and blithely continue to execute the experiment, trying to "do the best they could" to randomize fifteen thousand patients when they knew that, at best, they could randomize only a third of that number. That would have guaranteed a trial that was under-powered, i.e. with an unacceptably high type II error rate. Instead, they reconsidered the hypothesis and assumption of the sample size. They focused on the event rate of the trial. They knew that not many patients would die of a myocardial infarction (MI)—this was a major reason why the sample size computed by the statisticians was so large. However, they wondered, what would happen if they modified the endpoint, adding to the fatal MI component those patients with a nonfatal myocardial infarction. Since the total number of fatal and nonfatal myocardial infarctions was greater than the number of fatal myocardial infarctions alone, fewer patients could be followed to get a more frequent endpoint, and the sample size would be substantially reduced, In addition, the pathogenesis of nonfatal myocardial infarction was quite similar to that of fatal MI, so that it was expected that reductions in total cholesterol levels would reduce the number of nonfatal myocardial infarctions produced. Thus by changing the endpoint of the study, the investigators reduced the sample size to less than four thousand while remaining true to their study hypothesis. Good communication between the corps of the trial led to a favorable sample size outcome.

The "Good Enough for Them" Sample Size Approach

What happened in LRC is fortunately, an increasingly common occurrence. Schisms between sample size computation and resource availability are resolved by thoughtful scientists carefully reconsidering experimental programs during their design phase. However, in some experiments, little thought goes into the sample size considerations, as one investigator piggybacks onto the results of another investigator's preceding experimental result.

Consider an investigator who is studying the myocardial infarction model in animals. He notices that a previous investigator has demonstrated with 30 mice the efficacy of a compound to improve post-myocardial infarction heart structure. He wishes to repeat the experiment with a different but related medication. Since the first investigator was able to reject the null hypothesis based on thirty mice, this investigator plans to study thirty mice as well. After all, it worked for investigator. . . .

The difficulty with this approach is that it typically considers only the positive scenario. If the test statistic falls into the critical region, the investigator has essentially "gotten away with it." However, if the second investigator's study is negative, then what? Without any explicit consideration of power, the likelihood of a population (of mice) receiving benefit but producing a small sample without benefit is great. Even if benefit were apparent in the population, it is likely that, in this small sample, benefit would not be produced. Most likely the experiment can be interpreted not as negative but only as uninformative, because of inadequate power. Sample size computations must consider not just the type I error, but power as well. A nonsignificant test statistic from a concordantly executed trial in a low-power environment does not mean that the trial is negative—only that it is uninformative.

Efficacy Seduction

The perspicacious investigator will see that the sample size formulas 5.12 projected and 5.28 above reveal an interesting relationship between the sample size and the effect size. The sample size decreases as the square of the efficacy increases. This shows that a dramatic reduction in sample size can results from a modest increase in efficacy.

This relationship resonates with the physician-scientists, who believe strongly in the intervention's ability to have a beneficial impact[3] on patients. In fact, this relationship is sometimes taken as an encouragement to make an even bolder statement about the

---

[3] Chapter 6 discusses the destructive power of these strong, untested belief systems.

effect of the intervention. Increasing the effectiveness of the intervention from, for example a 20 percent reduction in event rate to a 30 percent reduction seems to increase the healing power of the intervention, and simultaneously permits a smaller sample size with its lower cost and administrative burden.

This seductive line of reasoning is quite misleading. Increasing the efficacy with the sole purpose of reducing the sample size blinds the investigator to moderate efficacy estimates that would potentially be clinically important. The investigator is blinded, since he would find moderate reductions in event rates that would have clinical import, but would not lead to statistically significant effects. For example, consider an experiment in which the investigator believes he has a therapy that reduces the occurrence of stroke in patients at risk for stroke. His sample size computation is based on a type I error of 0.10, power of 85 percent, and a cumulative stroke mortality rate of 0.25 in the placebo group. He believes the therapy will reduce the cumulative stroke rate from 0.25 to 0.20, a 20 percent reduction. This computation reveals a sample size of 3,628. However, he sees from formula 5.28 that by assuming a 35 percent reduction in stroke (leading to a cumulative stroke event rate of 0.163) he has reduced the sample size from 3,628 to 1,103, a 70 percent reduction!

The experiment is concordantly executed, in which 552 patients are randomized each of the two groups: placebo therapy or active therapy. The reduction in sample size is well earned if 138 (25 percent) of the patients in the placebo have a stroke, and ninety (16.3 percent) of the patients in the active group have a stroke. However, what if there are not ninety but 116 deaths in the active group (for a cumulative stroke rate of 0.210). The efficacy is $(0.25 - 0.21)/0.25 = 16$ percent. Now, an intervention that produces a 16 percent reduction in stroke mortality may be of great interest to the medical community. Unfortunately, however, this investigator cannot provide sufficient reassurance that this 16 percent finding is not just a product of sampling error (i.e., a type I error). The sample size is so small that the investigator cannot discern this effect "signal" from the background "noise" of sampling error. Even though the finding is clinically relevant, it is statistically insignificant.

This scenario is often the basis of the advice not to overestimate therapy effectiveness. It is often wisest to set efficacy in the lower interval in which there is clinical interest.

However, there is a power dividend

We have seen that it is dangerous to assume an unrealistically large estimate of efficacy solely to minimize the sample size requirment of the experiment. This is a common problem in clinical experiments involving equivalence. It is easy to not reject the null hypothesis for small sample sizes, but without adequate power to protect from sampling error, we cannot conclude that these experiments are negative. Consider an experiment designed to establish the efficacy of a medication in patients with severe ischemic heart disease. Patients will be randomized to either placebo therapy or the intervention, and followed for five years. The investigator computes a sample size based on equation 5.28 using a two-sided alpha of 0.075 and a power of 80 percent, to detect a 30 percent reduction in total mortality from the placebo group cumulative mortality rate of 35 percent. The trial size is 516 patients, 258 each for the placebo and treatment group.

The implications of this design are somewhat subtle but important to examine. A 35 percent event rate in the placebo group translates to ninety-one placebo deaths during the course of the trial. If the investigator is correct and there is a 30 percent reduction from this cumulative mortality rate in the active group, then he can expect a $(0.70)(0.35) = 0.245$ cumulative mortality rate or 64 deaths in the treatment group. What would the test statistic be if these predictions proved to be correct? A quick computation reveals that the test statistic is 2.59 and the two sided p value is 0.01.

How did this happen? The investigator had calculated the sample size based on a two sided alpha of 0.075. Why is the test statistic based on the assumption so much more extreme? Power. From equation 3, we can compute the size of the test statistic required for 80 percent power. The equation is.

$$1 - \beta = P\left[N(0,1) > Z_{1-\alpha/2} - \frac{\Delta}{\sqrt{var[p_x - p_y]}}\right] \tag{5.33}$$

which for this problem becomes

$$0.80 = p[N(0,1) > 1.775 - \text{Test statistic}]$$

revealing that the value of the test statistic is 2.61, close to the 2.59 obtained if the experiment was executed per protocol, and the protocol assumptions were realized in the sample.

The implications are immediate. If the designed efficacy reveals a p value of 0.01, then adequately powering an experiment allows for smaller efficacies to be considered statistically significant as well. Thus efficacies less than 30 percent would still fall in the critical region. A simple computation shows that efficacy of 20 percent and higher would be statistically significant. The consideration of power reveals a range of efficacies which would lead to rejection of the null hypothesis. It is the job of the investigator to match this range with the efficacies for which there is critical interest. The best advice is not to over estimate efficacy. Design the trial to detect modest clinical efficacy.

Conclusions

Power and p values are intertwined. This interrelationship can lead to danger for the unwary trial designer. Forcing type I error to extremely low levels will suck the power from the experiment. Sample size computations provided here show how to incorporate type I and type II error concerns into an experiment. However, the sample size computation, although composed only of mathematics, often is subject to the strong persistent undertow exerted by the resource centers of a clinical experiment. This is appropriate, and dialogue between all involved parties should be frank and open, for the good of the trial. Once the experiment is under way, discordance concerns preclude major changes in sample size goals. Therefore, honest discussion of logistical and financial issues should be encouraged during the research program's design phase.

References

1. Lachim, J.M., (1981) "Introduction to sample size determinations and power analyses for clinical trials," *Controlled Clinical Trials* 2:93–114.
2. Sahai, H., and Khurshid, A., (1996) "Formulae and tables for determination of sample size and power in clinical trials for testing differences in proportions for the two sample design," *Statistics in Medicine* 15:1–21.

3. Davy, S.J. and Graham, O.T., (1991) "Sample size estimation for comparing two or more treatment groups on clinical trials," *Statistics in Medicine* 10:3–43.
4. Donner, A., (1984) "Approach to sample size estimation in the design of clinical trials — a review," *Statistics in Medicine* 3:199–214.
5. George S.L., and Desue, M.M., (1974) "Planning the size and duration of a clinical trial studying the time to some critical event," *Journal of Chronic Disease* 27:15–24.

6

"Sir, you are unethical!" One-tailed vs. Two-tailed Testing

"Sir, you are unethical!" No matter how firmly I stand on the rectitude of my professional beliefs in a debate, this verbal blast will knock my ego off its feet. It is a terrible thing to utter and to hear uttered. I don't think that I am alone in my reaction to what is for physicians scathing criticism. No greater character wound can be inflicted than "You are unethical!"

Ethical conduct does not play an important role in our work in health care—it plays the principal one. Ethics are present in every conversation we have with patients, in every treatment plan we formulate, and in each of our research efforts. Perhaps the issue of test sidedness in a clinical experiment is a technical matter for mathematical statisticians, but for health care workers it is an issue of ethics. Test sidedness goes to the heart of the patient and community protection responsibilities of physicians. Decisions concerning test sidedness precisely define the battleline where our deep seated belief in therapy effectiveness collides with our obligatory prime concern for patient welfare.

Evidence Strength vs. Belief Strength

The attraction of one-sided (benefit only) testing begins with the earliest introduction to statistics in medicine. Many workers, after concluding an introductory section in significance testing, come away with the idea that the one-tailed (benefit only) test is efficient, and that two-tailed tests are wasteful. Consider the example of a test statistic which falls on the benefit side of a two sided critical region. It is very tempting to argue that the evidence seems clear. The test statistic is positive—why continue to insist on placing alpha in the negative, opposite side of the distribution? Be adaptive, be flexible, they would say. Respond to the persuasive nature of the data before you. Clearly the test statistic falls in the upper tail—the benefit tail—of the probability distribution. That is where the efficacy measure is. That is where the magnitude of the effect will be measured. Place your alpha there, like a flag in a new and promising land.

We want to discover benefit. This is why we are in research. Physician do not like to harbor the notion that the interventions we have developed for the benefit of our patients can do harm. Unfortunately, harm is often done. Well meaning physicians, through ignorance, injure their patients commonly. The use of cutting and bleeding in earlier centuries and the use of potent purgatives in this century are only two of the most notorious examples.

Do we as physicians take our responsibilities to our patients too seriously? No—but we must continually recognize what for us is so often unrecognizable—the possibility that we may have harmed others. The fact that a physician believes in a therapy does not make that therapy right. We may believe in a therapy and be wrong. Making our belief vehement only makes us vehemently wrong. Physicians must therefore remain ever vigilant for hazard of patient harm: the more strongly we believe in the benefit of a therapy, the more we must protect our patients, their families, and our communities from the harm our actions may inadvertently cause. The two-sided test shines bright, direct light on our darkest unspoken fears—that we as physicians and health care workers, despite our best efforts, might do harm.

Physicians often develop strongly held beliefs because of the forces of persuasion we must bring to bear when we discuss options with patients. We find ourselves in the position of advocating therapy choices for patients who rely heavily on our recommendations and opinions. We often must appeal to the better nature of patients who are uncertain in their decisions. We must be persuasive. We learn to use a combination of tact, firmness, and prestige to convince patients of the best approach in managing their health problems. We may feel too strongly about some therapy options, but certainly ambivalence is much worse.

Patient decisions may involve second opinions, but they are the opinions of other physicians, again vehemently expressed. Perhaps the day will come when physicians will be dispassionate dispensers of information about therapy choices but today is not that day.

The force behind vehement physician opinion can be magnified by the additional energy required to initiate and drive a study program. In research, enthusiasm is required to carry forward a joint effort. The proponents of the intervention must persuade their colleagues that the experiment is worthy of their time and labor. The investigators must convince sponsors (private or public) that the experiment is worth doing, and their argument often includes a forcefully delivered thesis on the prospects for the trial's success. This is necessary, since sponsors, who often must choose among a collection of proposed experiments, are understandably more willing to underwrite trials with a greater chance of demonstrating benefit. It is difficult to lobby for commitments of hundreds of thousands, if not millions of dollars, to gain merely an "objective appraisal of the intervention's effect". People invest dollars for success. In this tempestuous environment, the principal investigator must fight the persistent undertow to become the therapy's adamant advocate.

The one-tailed (benefit only) test is all too near at hand for these strong advocates. The investigators believe the therapy will work, and sometimes they unconciously allow themselves to imperceptibly drift away from the real possibility of harm befalling their patients. The one sided (benefit only) significance test has the allure of being consistent with their belief and providing some statistical efficiency. This is the great trap.

UMPTs

We have pointed out earlier that there is no mathematical preference for one level of type I error over another. The level of alpha is arbitrary and the mathematical foundation for significance testing is not strengthened or vitiated with the choice of a particular type I error rate. However, the case is different for choosing the sidedness of a significance test. In a strictly mathematical sense, the justification for the one-tailed (benefit only) test is slightly stronger than that for two sided testing. This argument is based solely on the criteria statisticians use to choose from among a host of competing statistical tests.

Let's consider first how to choose among several estimators of an effect. How should one best use the data obtained from a sample of patients to estimate a parameter, e.g., a cumulative event rate? The prospect of carrying out persuasive statistical inference is not promising if we cannot agree on the best way to use the data to compute the event rate. Therefore we must have some rules for choosing from a collection of competing estimators of a population parameter.[1] In the simplist case of deciding upon the best estimator for μ, the population mean of a normal distribution, why have we settled upon the sample mean, which we compute as $\sum_{i=1}^{n} x_i \Big/ n$? Why not some other quantity?

When constructing new estimates for a parameter, statisticians recognize that many competing estimators are available. Statisticians have developed properties that can be useful in discriminating between a host of estimators. One important property is unbiasdness. If, over many samples, the average of the estimator is the parameter, then the estimate is unbiased; the estimator does not overestimate more than it underestimates. Another characteristic of a good estimator is consistency. As the sample gets larger and larger, the estimator should get closer to the parameter. A third characteristic of the parameter is its variance—the smaller the variance, the more confidence we have that the estimate will close to the parameter. Each of these features is used to identify the best estimator.

Identifying estimators with a combination of these factors is critical. For example, the first, most natural estimator for the population variance from a sample of observations is $\sum_{i=1}^{n} (x_i - \bar{x})^2 \Big/ n$. However, statisticians quickly realized that this estimator, although consistent, was biased for estimating σ^2 and, if used, would underestimate the population variance. For this reason the related but unbiased estimator $s^2 = \sum_{i=1}^{n} (x_i - \bar{x})^2 \Big/ (n-1)$ is used.

Even with these standards of bias, consistency, and variance, can statisticians ever be assured that they have identified the best

[1] In general, estimators based on the sample data are used to estimate parameters in a population. Thus the sample mean is the estimator used to estimate the population mean, a number that is unobserved.

estimator? For example, can we ever be assured that, using these standards of judgments, statisticians will not identify another estimator for μ, the population mean of a normal distribution which is also unbiased, consistent, and has a smaller variance than $\sum_{i=1}^{n} x_i \big/ n$? In most cases in statistics, there is no such assurance. However, there is a collection of theorems which state that, if one has an estimator which meets certain properties, that estimator cannot be improved—no better unbiased estimator can ever be found. These unique estimators are called uniformly minimum variance unbiased estimators (UMVUE). As the name suggests, UMVUE's are unbiased and have been proven to have the smallest possible variance. The proof that an estimator is UMVUE is a singular event in its development because the proof is a promise that no other unbiased candidate will outperform it. Examples include the sample mean as an estimate for the population mean from a normal distribution. Another example is the least square estimates of coefficient parameters defined in regression analyses[2]. An analogous situation exists with hypothesis testing. For a given testing circumstance, there may be many imaginable ways to construct a significance test for a null and alternative hypothesis. How does one decide which is best? Tests are compared by first keeping alpha constant, and then computing for each test the probability that it will reject the null hypothesis when the alternative hypothesis is true[3]. The test that has the greatest power is preferred. However, as is the case with estimators there are a class of tests which are uniformly most powerful (UMP). That is, a UMP significance test has the greatest probability of rejecting the null hypothesis when the alternative hypothesis is true for a given alpha level, i.e. computing each test's power. Like UMVU estimators, uniformly most powerful tests are rare, but desirable.

When does a UMP test exist? When working with commonly used distributions (e.g., the normal distribution, exponential distribution, Poisson distribution, binomial distribution), one-sided significance tests concerning the parameters of these distributions are UMP tests. The two-sided tests are not UMP precisely because the type I error has to be apportioned across the two tails. Allo-

---

[2] An important caveat in regression analysis is that the estimators must be linear functions of the dependent variable.

[3] This is the definition of power, which will be discussed in more detail in chapter 6.

cating type I error in each tail when the test statistic from any one experiment can fall in only one tail engenders an inefficiency in the significance test. Thus, strictly from an optimality perspective, the one-tailed test is superior.

Knowledge vs. Faith

However, are statistically optimal tests the best criterion? Are they of necessity clinically ethical? This is an issue where the tension between the mathematics and the ethics of clinical research is high. One-tailed (benefit only) testing speaks to our intuition as researchers. We believe we know the tail in which the test statistic will fall. Why not put all of the type I error there? The one sided test resonates with our own belief in the effectiveness of the therapy. We have experience with the therapy, and have recognized patients in which it works well and patients in which it doesn't. We may have even come to rely on the therapy in our practices. Why place alpha in the tail of the distribution in which the test statistic will not fall? We are convinced of the importance of managing Type I error. Why choose to waste it now? Why should we allocate Type I error for an event that we do not believe will occur?

The operative word here is *believe*. The best experimental designs have their basis in knowledge—not faith. Research design requires that we separate our beliefs from our knowledge about the therapy. We are *convinced* of the intervention's efficacy, but we do not *know* the efficacy. We accept the therapy because of what we have seen in practice, however our view is not objective, but skewed. We may have seen only those patients who would have improved regardless of the therapy. Those patients who did not respond to therapy may have involved themselves in additional therapy without our knowledge. As convincing as our platform is, it provides only a distorted view of the true effect of the intervention in the community. We may believe strongly, but our vantage point as practicing physicians assures us that we have not seen clearly. Admitting the necessity of the trial is a first important acknowledgment that the investigator does not know what the outcome will be. Therefore, an important requirement in the design of an experiment is that the investigators separate their beliefs from their information. The experiment should be designed based on *knowledge of* rather than *faith in* the therapy.

There are many remarkable singular examples of the surprises that await physician scientist who are not careful with the tails of the distribution. Two notorious ones follow.

The arrhythmia suppression hypothesis and CAST

The "arrhythmia suppression" theory is an example of the difficulties that occur when decisions for patient therapy at the community level are based on untested physician belief rather than on tried and tested fact.[4]

In the middle of this century, there began an understanding among cardiologists that heart arrhythmias were not uniform, but instead depicted a spectrum with well-differentiated mortality prognoses. Some of these rhythms, such as premature atrial contractions and premature ventricular contractions, were in and of themselves benign. Others, such as ventricular tachycardia, were dangerous. Ventricular fibrillation, in which vigorous, coordinated ventricular contractions were reduced to amorphic, wormy, non-contractile, uncoordinated ventricular muscle movement led to immediate death. The appearance of these dangerous rhythms was often unpredictable; however, they occurred more commonly in the presence of atherosclerotic cardiovascular disease and, more specifically, were often present after a myocardial infarction. Drugs had been available to treat heart arrhythmias, but many of these (e.g., quinidine and procainamide) produced severe side effects and were difficult for patients to tolerate. However, scientists were developing a newer generation of drugs (e.g., ecanide, flecanide, and moritzacine) that produced fewer side effects.

The effectiveness and safety of these newer drugs were examined in a collection of case series studies. As the number of patients placed on these drugs increased, the sense was that patients with dangerous arrhythmias who took them were showing some reversal of these deadly heart rhythms and perhaps some clinical improvement. However, the absence of a control group makes case series studies notoriously difficult to assess. When patients survived, their survival was often attributed to drug therapy.

---

[4] Much of this section is taken from Thomas Moore's book *Deadly Medicine.*

However, patient deaths are often not counted against the therapy being tested. When the patient died, investigators suggested that the patient was just too sick to survive, i.e. no drug could have helped the patient. However despite some debate, a consensus arose that patient survival was also improved.

The consensus that these newer drugs were having a beneficial impact on arrhythmia suppression, and perhaps on mortality gained momentum as prestigious physicians lent their imprimatur to the arrhythmia suppression hypothesis. The sponsors of these drugs, along with established experts in cardiology and cardiac rhythm disturbances, continued to present data to the federal Food and Drug Administration (F. D. A.), applying pressure on that regulatory body to approve the drugs for use by practicing physicians. This body of evidence presented did not contain a randomized controlled clinical trial to test the efficacy of these compounds only case series. However, after persistent lobbying, advisory committee deliberations, and extensive discussions both publicly and privately, the F. D. A. relented and approved the new antiarrhythmic agents. As a consequence of this approval, physicians began to prescribe the drugs not just to patients with severe rhythm disturbances, but also to patients with very mild arrhythmias. This expanded use was consistent with the growing consensus that these drugs were also beneficial in blocking the progression from mild heart arrhythmias to more serious rhythm disturbances. The F. D. A. was extremely uncomfortable with this untested evolution in usage because it had not forseen it, but was powerless to limit the use of the drugs. Soon, many of the nation's physicians were using the drug to treat the relatively mild ventricular arrhythmia of premature beats.

However, there were researchers who were interested in putting the arrhythmia suppression hypothesis to the test. Working with the National Institutes of Health (NIH), they designed an experiment called CAST (Cardiac Arrhythmia Suppression Trial) that would randomize almost 4,400 patients to one of these new antiarrhythmic agents or placebo and follow them over time. This experiment would be double blind, so that neither the physicians administering the drug nor patients taking the drug would know whether the agent they were taking was active. Clinical trial specialists designed this experiment with established, prolific experience in clinical trial methodology. These workers computed that 450 deaths would be required for them to establish the effect of the therapy. However, they designed the trial as one-sided, anticipating that only therapy benefit would result from this research effort. As designed, the trial would not be stopped because the therapy was harmful, only for efficacy or the lack of promise of the trial to show efficacy. This was an amazing decision. See Thomas Moore *Deadly Medicine* (page 203–204)

> The CAST investigators ... wanted a structure that eliminated the possibility of ever proving that the drugs were harmful, even by accident. If the drugs were in fact harmful, convincing proof would not occur because the trial would be halted when the chances of proving benefit had become too remote.

The fact that the investigators designed the trial as one-sided, reveals the degree to which they believed the therapy would reduce mortality. However, although CAST was designed as a one sided hypothesis test by its investigators, the Data and Safety Monitoring Board[5] insisted on reviewing the data without knowledge of the actual treatment group, with significance test at the 0.025 level. This was tantamount to a two sided hypothesis test for the interim data review. However, the board did not overtly contradict the investigators' desire that this should be a test for benefit.

During CAST recruitment, many in the practicing medical community viewed the trial with comtempt. Clinicians were already using these drugs to suppress premature ventricular contractions. Why was a clinical trial needed? Hadn't the F. D. A. already approved these new antiarrhythmic agents? Hadn't numerous editorials published by distinguished scientists in well-respected journals magnified the benefits of this therapeutic approach? Why do an expensive study at this point? Furthermore, why would a physician who believed in this therapy agree to enter her patients into a clinical trial where there was a fifty-fifty chance that the patient would receive placebo therapy? Vibrant discussions and contentious exchanges occurred during meetings of physicians in which CAST representatives exhorted practicing physicians to recruit their patients into the study. At the conclusion of a presentation by a CAST recruiter, a physician, clearly angry, rose and said of the trial recruiter, "You are immoral," contending that it was improper to deny this drug to half of the randomized participants [1].

However, before recruitment ended, CAST scientists tabulated

---

[5] The Data and Safety Monitoring Board (DSMB) is an august group of distinguished scientists, not directly affiliated with the trial, who review all of the data in an unblinded review of the experiment's results. They can decide to stop a trial prematurely if it shows early benefit or unanticipated harm.

important differences. After one third of the required number of patients were recruited for the study, the data analysis provided shocking results. Out of the 730 patients randomized to the active therapy, 56 died. Of the 725 patients randomized to placebo there were 22 deaths. In a trial designed to demonstrate only the benefit of antiarrhythmic therapy, this therapy was discovered to be almost four times as likely to kill patients as placebo. In this one-tailed experiment the "p value" was 0.0003, in the "other tail"

The investigators reacted to these devastating findings with shock and disbelieve. They had embraced the arrhythmia suppression hypothesis, to the point where they had excluded all possibility of identifying a harmful effect. It was difficult to recruit patients to this study because so many practicing physicians believed in suppressing premature ventricular contractions. Yet the findings of the experiment proved them wrong. There has been much debate on the implications of CAST for the development of antiarrhythmic therapy. However, an important lesson is that physicians cannot form conclusions about population effects by extrapolating their own beliefs.

Lipid Research Clinics Results

CAST was an example of investigators' surprise at finding harm in the face of full expectation of therapy benefit. The issue in the Lipid Research Clinic (LRC) study was one of efficacy. For these investigators, not even a one-tailed test was sufficient to insure success.

The Lipid Research Clinics study was an examination of the role of cholesterol reduction therapies in reducing the risk of clinical events. Designed in the 1970s by lipidologists working in concert with experienced clinical trial methodologists, the LRC trial set out to establish with some finality the importance of cholesterol level reduction in reducing clinical sequelae of atherosclerotic cardiovascular disease. It was designed to randomize patients either to cholesterol reduction therapy or to no therapy, and then to follow these patients over time, counting the number of fatal and nonfatal myocardial infarctions that occurred. LRC required over 3,500 patients to be followed for seven years to reach its conclusion, incorporated into a pre-specified hypothesis test. The final trial test statistic would be assessed using a prospectively declared one-sided hypothesis test at the 0.01 level. If the resulting z-score at the trial's conclusion was greater than 2.33, the investigators would conclude that the therapy was beneficial.

The investigators did not underestimate the importance of their work. They knew the field was contentious, and that their study would be criticized regardless of its findings. The investigators designed the protocol with great deliberation and care. Upon its completion, they converted their lucid protocol into a design manuscript, publishing it in the prestigious *Journal of Chronic Diseases*[3]. This was a praiseworthy effort. The investigators prospectively and publicly announced the goals of the research effort and, more importantly, disseminated the rules by which they would decide the success or failure of the experiment for all to review before the data were collected and tabulated. This is one of the best approaches to reducing experimental discordance.

In 1984, the study's conclusion were anticipated with great excitement. When published in the *Journal of the American Medical Association* [4] they revealed that active therapy produced an 8.5 percent reduction in cholesterol. Furthermore, there were 19 percent fewer nonfatal myocardial infarctions and 24 percent fewer deaths from cardiovascular disease in the active group. These differences were announced as statistically significant, and the investigators determined the trial to be positive. The final Z-score was 1.92. The P value was less than 0.05!?!

How was this possible? The critical region for the hypothesis test was $Z > 2.33$. Since the achieved z-score of 1.92 did not fall in this critical region, the study should have been considered negative by the LRC investigators' own criteria,. Yet the investigators concluded that the experiment was positive. Their rationale was that the significance test should now be interpreted not as a one-tailed test with a significance level of 0.01, as was planned and announced, but as a one sided test at the 0.05 level. This adjustment changed the critical region to be $Z > 1.645$.

They changed the significance level of the test, based on the findings of the trial! The fact that the investigators published a design manuscript prospectively, highlighting the rules by which the trial would be judged and the standards to which the trial should be held, makes the change in the required test significance level singularly ignoble. It is hard to find a clearer example of alpha corruption[6] than this.

---

[6] See chapter 1.

As we might expect, there are many plausible explanations for the diluted finding of efficacy for LRC. The cholesterol reduction therapy chosen for the trial, cholestyramine, was difficult for patients to tolerate. This difficulty led to fewer patients taking the medication, vitiating the measured effectiveness of the compound. It must be said that, even with this weak cholesterol reduction effect, the investigators were able to identify a trend for a reduction in morbidity and mortality associated with cholestyramine. The study produced much new information, which would have served as a firm, scientifically based foundation for the next clinical experiment. However, the investigators chose instead to fly in the face of their own prospective rules for assessing the strength of evidence in their study, resulting not in illumination, but in withering criticism from the scientific community. The LRC investigators had too little objective evidence to believe in the cholesterol reduction hypothesis as strongly as they did at the trial's inception. They believed in it to the point of excluding a formal examination for the presence of a harmful effect of cholestyramine,[7] choosing instead a one sided (benefit only) evaluation. This belief also led them to take the astounding step of corrupting their study when the type I error appeared larger than they anticipated. Rather than bolster the cholesterol reduction hypothesis, perhaps refining it for the next study, their alpha corrupting maneuver besmirched it. The one-sided test was a symptom of "strong belief disease."

In health care, time and again, well-meaning researchers identify an intervention they believe will be effective in alleviating suffering and perhaps prolonging life. This noble, and the raison-d'être of medical research. Unfortunately, all too often the fervor of this belief spills over, tainting the design and execution of an experiment in order to demonstrate efficacy. These experiments are often encumbrances to medical progress rather than bold steps forward. The one-tailed test is not the ultimate problem; it is the symptom of untested investigator beliefs masquerading as truth.

Sample Size Issues

Another argument raised in defense of one-sided testing is sample size efficiency. With concern for only one of the two tails of the

---

[7] There was concern that cholesterol redution was associated with violent death.

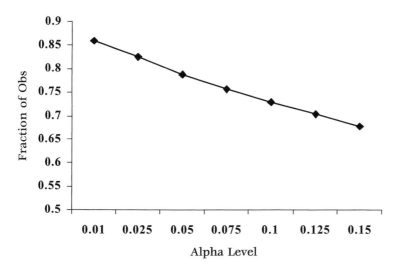

This graph depicts the fraction of observations in a two sided test required for a one tailed test. Assumes the trial is designed to detect a 20% reduction in endpoint events from a control group cumulative event rate of 25% with 80% power

Figure 6.1. Fraction of Observations in a Two Tailed Test Required for a One Tailed Test

probability distribution, one might naturally expect there to be a substantial reduction in the size of the sample, since the one sided test focuses on only one tail of the probability distribution of effect. However, although the savings are apparent, they do not occur at the level one might expect. Figure 6.1 depicts the relationship between the fraction of observations needed in a two-tailed test that are required in a one-tailed test, from the design of a randomized clinical experiment where the goal is to demonstrate a 20 percent reduction in clinical event rates from a cumulative control group event rate of 25 percent with 80 percent power.

If we would expect that 50 percent of the observations required for a two-sided test were needed for a one-tailed significance test in this example, then the curve would reveal a flat line at y = 0.50 for the different levels of alpha. The curve in figure 6.1 demonstrates something quite different. For example, for an alpha level of 0.075, 76 percent of the observations required in the two-tailed test are needed for the one-sided test. At any level of alpha examined, the 50 percent value is not achieved. Although some savings are evident, the number of required observation for a one-tailed test are more than 50 percent of that necessary for the two sided test. The sample size savings for the one-tailed test are much smaller than one might naively expect.

Hoping for the Best, Preparing for the Worst

There are important limitations in carrying out a one-tailed test in a clinical research effort. In my view, the major difficulty is that the one sided testing philosophy reveals a potentially dangerous level of investigator consensus that there is no possibility of patient harm produced by the intervention being tested. As we have seen in CAST, this sense of invulnerability to harm can ambush well-meaning investigators, delivering them over to stupefaction and confusion as they struggle to assimilate the unexpected, devastating results of their efforts. We physicians don't like to accept the possibility that, well meaning as we are, we may be hurting the patients we work so hard to help; however, a thoughtful consideration of our history persuades us that this is all to often the case. The intelligent application of the two-tailed test requires deliberate efforts to consider the possibility of patient harm during the design phase of the experiment. This concern, expressed early and formally in the trial's design, can be very naturally translated into effective steps taken during the course of the experiment. In circumstances where the predesign clinical intuition is overwhelmingly in favor of a finding of benefit, the investigators should go out of their way to assert what level of alpha will provide community level protection from harm in the research program. It is fine to hope for the best, as long as we prepare for the worst.

However, the use of a two-sided test does not in and of itself guarantee adequate community level protection. In these circumstances, the investigators' mandate for alpha allocation extends beyond the simple stipulation that significance testing be two-tailed.

Symmetrics vs. Ethics

Once we have made the decision in the design phase of an experiment for a two-tailed significance test, we very naturally and easily divide alpha into two equal components placing half in the tail signifying harm and half in the benefit tail of the probability distribution. This assumption of the symmetric allocation of alpha is perhaps the easiest assumption to justify, but locks us into a re-flexive choice involving a community protection issue. It would be useful to examine other options.

Consider for example, an investigation of the treatment of diabetes mellitus. Diabetes, in addition to its serious renal, micro-vasculature, lens and retinal complications, is a well known risk factor for atherosclerotic heart disease. Patients with diabetes mellitus have a greater risk for atherosclerotic disease. However, the debate over the control of adult onset (type II) diabetes melli-tus has persisted for several decades. Should blood glucose be strictly monitored and confined to a narrow range (tight control), or should it be allowed a more broad range of excursion? Suppose an investigator is interested in determining if the tight control of adult onset diabetes mellitus can reduce the risk of death due to cardiovascular disease.

The investigator believes that the risk of cardiovascular disease in the community of type II diabetics can be reduced by 20 per-cent with the tight control of diabetes. He plans the following ex-periment. Select a random sample of patients suffering from adult onset diabetes from the population at large, randomly allocating them to either standard control or tight control, and follow these patients for five years, counting the number of cardiovascular deaths in each group.

The investigator believes that the tight control group will expe-rience fewer cardiovascular events, but he is also interested in protecting his community. He acknowledges, that, despite his be-lief, the result might not be what he expects. Appropriately sepa-rating his belief from his information, he designs a two-sided test. A test statistic that appears in the extreme higher tail of the nor-mal distribution would suggest benefit; one in the lower tail would suggest harm. He does not expect harm to occur as a result of the tight control, but he prepares for it.

This strategy is consistent with the points we have made earlier in this chapter, but is it sufficient? In order to decide in favor of benefit, the investigator needs a cardiovascular event rate to be 20 percent less in the tight control group than in the standard control group. However, must the tight control intervention be associated with 20 percent greater cardiovascular mortality before the inves-tigator will conclude that tight control is harmful? Is this sym-metric approach of strength of evidence in line with the oath to "first do no harm"? The symmetry argument insures that the strength of evidence of harm is the same as that required to conclude benefit, but if the ethical concern is harm, perhaps less evidence of harm should be required. The "first do no harm" principle identifies protection as the primary issue. If we are to protect the patients, we must be especially vigilant for the possibility for harm. We must stop the trial if harm occurs, at the acceptable risk of placing new therapy development on hold. Unfortunately, therapy used for the treatment of type II diabetes mellitus has been associated with harm in the past.[8] Knowing this, the investigator must assure himself and his patients that he will remain vigilant for the possibility that the new method of diabetes control he is using is not harming his patients.

Consider the following alternative strategy for alpha allocation. Recognizing that his primary responsibility is to protect the community from a harmful effect of the tight control intervention, the investigator decides that a test statistic suggesting harm should not be as extreme the test statistic he would accept as suggesting benefit. As a first approximation for the overall alpha for the experiment, the investigator chooses alpha at 0.05. He apportions 0.03 of this alpha in the harm tail of the distribution, and the remaining 0.02 in the benefit arm. This leads to the following decision rule.

Reject the null hypothesis in favor of harm if TS ≤ -1.88.
Reject the null hypothesis in favor of benefit if TS ≥ -2.05.

The investigator's oath-mandated greater concern for the possibility that he is harming his patients is explicitly expressed in this significance testing. The sample size is chosen to be adequate for the tail of the distribution with the smallest alpha allocation.

Now, at the conclusion of the concordantly executed[9] trial, the test statistic is computed and is seen to be 2.18. What is the p value for the study?[10] It is the probability that a normal random variable is less than or equal to -1.88 plus the probability that a normal deviate is greater than 2.18 or $P[Z < -1.88] + P[Z > 2.18] = 0.03 + 0.015 = 0.045$. One would correctly conclude that this concordantly executed study is positive. Note that this p value construction is different from the traditional p value computation. Tra-

---

[8] See for example, the University Group Diabetes Project [4].
[9] Concordance is defined in chapter 1 as research which is executed according to its protocol with no data motivated changes in the analysis plan.
[10] Remember that alpha is apportioned before the study is executed, and p values are computed at the end of the study, based on the study data.

Table 6.1. Alpha Table: Trial Conclusion

Primary Endpoint	Alpha Allocation	Alpha Expenditure
Harm	0.030	0.030
Benefit	0.020	0.015
Total	0.050	0.045

ditionally with a test statistic of 2.18, the p value would be computed as

$$P[|Z| > 2.18] = p[Z < -2.18] + P[Z > 2.18]$$
$$= 2P[Z > 2.18] = (2)(0.015) = 0.030.$$

In this computation, the probability of a type I error is reduced from the pre-specified level of 0.05 not just on the benefit side of the distribution, but on the harm side as well. How is this justified? Why should we transmute the reduction of the possibility of type I error for benefit into a reduction in the possibility of the type I error for harm?[11] The only justification for this reduction in the harm arm of alpha is the a priori notion of symmetry. If the investigator at the trial's inception constructs the two-sided test as symmetrical, he is arguing that the alpha error be channeled symmetrically at the end of the experiment. His best guess at the inception of the study was at the 0.05 level, so he apportions alpha symmetrically as 0.025. At the conclusion of the experiment, although the type I error in the benefit arm decreased from 0.025 to 0.015, the *a priori* assumption of symmetry remains in force. The finding of 0.015 in the benefit side of the distribution results in a total alpha expenditure of 0.030.

However, with the removal of the symmetry constraint a priori, there is no longer justification for the symmetric construction of the p value. The possibility of a type I error for harm has not been updated by the experiment, and remains unchanged at 0.035. The estimate of the magnitude of type I error in the benefit portion of the efficacy distribution is decreased from 0.035 to 0.015, and the p value for the experiment is $0.030 + 0.015 = 0.045$.

It would be a mistake to view the results of this experiment as

---

[11] This is as opposed to the question, what is the location of the distribution of efficacy in the population based on the test statistic, which is a Bayesian question.

Table 6.2. Asymmetric Alpha Allocation: Total Alpha = 0.125

Primary Endpoint	Alpha Allocation
Harm	0.10
Benefit	0.025
Total	0.125

Table 6.3. Alpha Table: Trial Conclusion (Test statistic = 2.18)

Primary Endpoint	Alpha Allocation	Alpha Expenditure
Harm	0.10	0.10
Benefit	0.025	0.0125
Total	0.125	0.1125

barely significant, as is often done in the reflexive 0.05 paradigm. The use of asymmetry has complicated the interpretation.

Let's return to the design phase of this argument to explore one other consideration. One could make a case that, given the strength of evidence so far suggesting the possibility of long-term harm of the treatment of diabetes, even more alpha should be evidence for harm. One possible allocation for alpha would be as in Table 6.2.

In this scheme, the overwhelming ethical concern is to identify the possibility of harm. The total alpha for the experiment is 0.125, but only 0.025 is identified for benefit. In this circumstance, the test statistic must be larger than 1.96 to demonstrate evidence of benefit, but only -1.28 to demonstrate evidence of harm.

Suppose now that the test statistic is observed as 2.18 Table 6.3. Then the experiment is positive and the total alpha expended $P[Z < -1.28] + P[Z > 2.18] = 0.10 + 0.015 = 0.115$.

The study should be viewed as positive for benefit since the total alpha allocated is less than the alpha allocated at the trial's beginning. Also, adequate population protection was provided for harm. Critics of the study who would minimize the findings of this trial should be reminded that the alpha for significance for benefit $= P[Z > 2.18] = 0.015$, suggesting sampling error is an unlikely explanation of the research findings.[12] However, the over-

---

[12] Of course the sample size, effect size, and its variability must also be assessed independently.

riding concern for population protection demanded the prospectively specified, asymmetric critical region.

In this case, the investigators have allocated alpha prospectively and intelligently, requiring sufficient strength of evidence for benefit while vigorously exercising their mandate for community protection. Nevertheless, many will feel uncomfortable about this nonstandard scheme for alpha allocation. We must keep in mind that the allocation the investigators have chosen stands on good ground, adhering to the following requirements, necessary and sufficient for its clear interpretation. First, alpha is allocated prospectively, in great detail. Secondly, the protocol involved the random selection of subjects from the population and the random allocation of therapy. Finally, the experiment was executed concordantly with no consequent alpha corruption. The investigators have wielded their mandate handsomely, providing adequate community protection while insisting on the same standard of efficacy required by the more traditional scientific community. The experimental findings would be reduced only in the eyes of those with a reflexive requirement of 0.05 with symmetric tails.

Conclusion

I believe one-tailed (benefit only) testing reflects a mind-set of physicians and health care researchers who believe their intervention can produce no harm, a philosophy which has been shown repeatedly to be faulty, and dangerous to patients and their families. Investigators who agree to the one-tailed (benefit only) approach to significance testing in a clinical experiment have closed parts of their minds to the possibility of harm entering into an avoidable flirtation with danger. In this sense, the one-tailed test is not the disease, it is only a symptom.

We as physicians and health care workers feel strongly about the treatment programs we advocate. This is required in our profession. However, these strong feelings often betray us since our day to day experience does not provide an objective view of the treatments. We need every tool we can find to help us gain that objective vantage point. The use of a two-sided significance test is of utmost importance. A forceful, intelligent argument for ethics will argue not only for a two-sided test, but asymmetrical allocation of alpha. Prospective identification of alpha is again critical here, and community protection predominates all other concerns. A sensitive, perceptive, ethical approach to alpha allocation for sidedness can complicate experimental design, but complexity in the name of ethics is no vice.

References

1. The CAST Investigators, (1989) "Preliminary Report: effect of encainide and flecainide on mortality in a randomized trial of arrhythmia suppression after myocardial infarction," *N Engl J Med* 321:406–412.
2. The Lipid Research Clinic Investigators, (1984) "The Lipid Research Clinics Program: Coronary Primary Prevention Trial Results," *Journal of the American Medical Association* 251:351–374.
3. The Lipid Research Clinic Investigators (1979) "The Lipid Research Clinics Program: "The Coronary Primary Prevention Trial; Design and Implementation," *Journal of Chronic Diseases* 32:609–631.
4. The UGDP Investigators, (1971) "University groups diabetes program: A study of the effect of hypoglycemic agents on vascular complications in patients with adult-onset diabetes," *Journal of the American Medical Association* 218:1400–1410.

7

CHAPTER

P Values and Multiple Endpoints I: Pernicious Abstractions?

In a large clinical trial, thousands and sometimes tens of thousands of patients are followed for years. This effort generates hundreds of thousands of data points, carefully collected, verified, entered and analyzed by many workers, themselves committing thousands of hours to this task. Is all of this effort for just a single *p* value?

The view that this colossal effort generating one and only one *p* value for a hypothesis test has long since been discarded. Rising up to replace this approach is the multiple-arm, multiple-endpoint clinical trial. Rather than focus on two arms (treatment and control) and one endpoint, these complicated experiments may have several treatment arms (e.g., one arm for each of three doses of therapy and a control arm) and, in addition, several endpoints (e.g. total mortality, total hospitalizations, and quality of life). However, every step out of one problem is a step right into another. The creation of these complicated clinical experiments with their complexity of endpoints has created a new host of problems in significance testing. This chapter will provide motivation to an investigator facing not the hazard, but the opportunity of allocating type I error in an experiment involving several endpoints. We will also provide advice for the interpretation of clinical experiments whose experimentalists have made no prospective statements for alpha allocation. The direct computations to pursue for alpha allocation appear in chapter 8.

The Great Trap: Experimental Efficiency vs. Interpretative Parsimony

Significance testing focuses on decision making—its original motivation was to draw a single conclusion concerning a single effect. To accomplish this, one experiment would be concordantly executed,[1] producing one conclusion (such as therapy A yields a better clinical result than placebo). We are now comfortable with the type I error statements stemming from such an experiment. However, investigative circumstances have arisen in which the final results of the program involve not just one endpoint, but a collection of endpoints. For example, chapter six provided examples in which a concordantly executed experiment tested the ability of a compound to reduce the total mortality rate. However, in reality, more than just one variable reflecting the outcome of a patient would be measured. In addition to total mortality, the experiment might measure the incidence of fatal and nonfatal myocardial infarctions, the cumulative rate of hospitalizations during the course of the trial, and the rate of surgical procedures during the experiment. Each of these measures has clinical merit, and trial designers, in choosing the measures to be assessed at the experiment's conclusion, add more endpoints, yielding to clinical trial efficiency; the incremental cost of additional endpoints diminishes.

For example, consider an experiment designed to randomize thousands of patients from the population and then follow them for as long as five years to carry out a significance test on fatal and nonfatal myocardial infarction. Here, the additional effort to collect information on, for example, the frequency of unstable angina and the frequency of hospitalizations for cardiovascular disease is small. After all, the investigator is already going to the trouble and expense to recruit, randomize and follow this patient cohort. Why not measure as much as you can? As long as there is genuine scientific interest in measuring these additional endpoints and the protocol is expanded prospectively during the design phase of the trial[2] these additional measurements are seen to hold promise.

---

[1] Concordant execution is the carrying out of an experiment according to its protocol, without a databased change in the analysis plan (chapter 1).

[2] Prospective identification is required to insure that acceptable standards of collections and definitions of morbiity are developed, avoiding any discordancy issues (chapter 1).

There is also a strong epidemiologic motivation for multiple endpoints. Clinical trial findings are more persuasive if the results for the main endpoint are substantiated by findings for the additional endpoints. For example, a study designed to assess the effect of a compound to reduce total mortality in patients suffering from heart failure is strengthened if it also same study demonstrates that the intervention also reduces total hospitalizations for heart failure and increases patient exercise tolerance. The endpoints in such a study "speak with one voice" about the effect of the medication. This coherency adds to the cogency of the trial's contention for therapy benefit. Multiple endpoint measurements can also provide information about the mechanism by which the intervention acts (building up the causality argument by bolstering biologic plausibility component of the epidemiologic tenets of causality[3]). In addition the choice of multiple endpoints may include endpoints examined in related clinical trials and depending on the findings, add to a consistency-of-effect argument.[4]

Thus efficiency concerns and epidemiologic considerations combine to support the notion of multiple endpoints in a single study. At the end of the trial, there is irresistible temptation to carry out significance testing on these endpoints, testing which holds out great promise for strengthening the experiment's thesis — and herein lies a great trap. It can be exceedingly difficult to interpret these endpoint findings, which were so easily and conveniently measured. In fact, the absence of adequate alpha safeguards, can rise up and strangle this multi-headed experiment.

The concept of trial efficiency, aided by powerful epidemiologic arguments, supports the measurement of multiple endpoints. Significance testing, however, implies that the more testing you do, the more likely the commission of a type I error becomes. Significance testing concerns itself with neither efficiency nor with epidemiologic criteria of coherence, biologic plausibility, or consistency. Significance testing represents a different paradigm, but a necessary one that we must integrate into the trial result interpretation as well. Significance testing keeps track of decisions drawn from the data, adding to the type I error with each new decision. Consider an experiment with a prospectively set type I error bound of 0.075, in which the significance test for the first endpoint produces a p value of 0.05 and a significance test on a second endpoint has a p value of 0.06. One might conclude that

---

[3] Chapter 3.

[4] Another of the epidemiologic tenets of causality from chapter 3.

since each result is less than the alpha allocated prospectively, the findings for each of these endpoints is positive. However, the probability of making at least one type I error from these two decisions is computed to be $1 - (0.95)(0.94) = 0.107$[5]. What conclusion should we draw? We need guidelines here, but, unfortunately, they are often not available. It is in the interpretation of these secondary endpoints where the requirement of clinical trial efficiency drives head-on with the parsimony of significance testing.

Don't Ask, Don't Tell...

As a first step out of this dilemma, investigators often rank endpoints in the order of importance. The one chosen as the primary endpoint is the endpoint which is considered the justification of the experiment, representing the best measure on which to judge the effectiveness of therapy. The primary endpoint is used to supply the "positive" or "negative" characterization of the trial results; it is the axis around which the trial revolves. Much attention is appropriately paid to this endpoint. Sample size estimates are constructed based on it, and the investigators work hard to insure that it is objectively measured during the course of the experiment. However, customarily no ranking or alpha allocation is afforded the secondary endpoints[6]. With no additional ranking or alpha allocation, the investigators and the scientific community are uncertain as to how to judge the findings of these additional endpoints. Many times, the findings for these secondary endpoints are reported as only nominal p values (that is, the raw p value produced from each of the significance tests is interpreted as though it is the only significance test executed in the experiment; there is no consideration of the global type I error). Letting nominal p values determine by themselves the significance of the findings for these secondary endpoints is allowing the data to determine the decision rule, an approach which is clearly alpha corruptive[7]. The absence of a demand by the scientific com-

---

[5] This calculation is an application of formula 1 appearing later in this chapter.
[6] Sometimes endpoints are ranked as secondary or tertiary but rarely is this ranking used in a sensitive construction of global type I error.
[7] See chapter 1 for a definition an examples of the destructive effects of type I errror corruption.

munity for specific rules to judge secondary endpoints and the absence of investigator initiative in providing these allocations to the scientific community prospectively is tantamount to a "don't ask, don't tell" approach, leading to confusion in interpreting the results of the endpoints at the trial's conclusion.

It is therefore no wonder that surprising results from non-primary endpoints or other measures can throw an expensive experiment into disarray and controversy. Consider the findings of the U.S. Carvedilol program [1]. In this research endeavor carvedilol, a new medication for the treatment of congestive heart failure, was tested against placebo in a prospectively designed, double blind[8], randomized controlled clinical trial program. In this program, 1,197 patients were screened and 1,094 patients were selected for one of four protocols and then randomized to a treatment arm or placebo in the selected protocol. There were 398 total patients randomized to placebo and 696 to carvedilol. At the conclusion of approximately one year of follow-up, 31 deaths had occurred in the placebo group and 22 in the active group, resulting in a relative risk[9] of 0.65 and a p value less than 0.001. The program was terminated, and the investigators posited that, since total mortality was an objective of the carvedilol program, the beneficial effect of carvedilol on total mortality should compel the federal Food and Drug Administration (F. D. A.) to approve the drug as effective in reducing the incidence of total mortality in patients suffering from congestive heart failure.

Although the manuscript describing the results of the trial stated that patients were stratified into one of four treatment protocols [1, page 1350], the manuscript did not state the fact that each of these protocols had its own prospectively identified primary endpoint, and that total mortality was not a primary or a secondary endpoint for any of the trials! Three of the trials had exercise tolerance as a primary endpoint and measures of morbidity from congestive heart failure as secondary endpoints. Furthermore, a protocol-by-protocol delineation of the primary endpoint results was not included in the manuscript. Interrogation revealed that the finding for the prospectively defined primary

---

[8] Double blind means that neither the treating physician, nor the patient knew the medication could tell if the medication the patient was given was placebo or carvedilol. Such an approach reduces the bias a physician would be subject to in her assessment of the patient's progress and experiences.
[9] The relative risk is based on a Cox proportional hazards model, a detail which should not distract from the discussion.

endpoint in three of the four trials was $p > 0.05$ (non-significant). The fourth study had as its primary endpoint hospitalization for heart failure; the statistical analysis for this primary endpoint was $p < 0.05$. Each of these four studies had secondary endpoints that assessed congestive heart failure morbidity, some of which were nominally significant ($p < 0.05$), others not. As pointed out by Fisher [2], total mortality was not an endpoint of any of the four studies in the program. Thus a research effort that at first glance appeared to be a cohesive trial with a total mortality primary endpoint, was upon close inspection a post hoc combined analysis for a non-prospectively defined endpoint.

This discovery produced a host of problems for the experiment's interpretation. Pre-specification of the anticipated analysis in the protocol of a trial has been an accepted standard among clinical trial workers [3] and certainly must be included in a manuscript describing that trial's results. In addition, the non-reporting of nonsignificant endpoints in clinical trials has been criticized [4]. The scientific community expects, and clinical trial workers require that analyses be provided for all prospectively stated endpoints. The fact that the results of a program claiming major benefit did not specifically define and report the analysis of the primary endpoint is a serious deficiency in a manuscript that purports to describe the effects of therapy. Unfortunately, by violating these fundamental trial tenets, the Carvedilol investigators open themselves up to the criticism that they selected the total mortality analysis because of its favorable results, thus biasing the conclusions and tainting the research effort to answer important scientific and clinical questions. The interpretation of this discordant program was both complex and contentions [2,5,6,7]. Unanticipated surprise findings on nonprimary endpoints can weaken rather than strengthen a trial.

As another example of the problems secondary endpoints can cause, consider the following hypothetical program. A randomized, controlled clinical trial is concordantly executed with a prospectively defined primary endpoint, P1, and three prospectively defined secondary endpoints, S1, S2 and S3. The only prospective statement was that a two-sided 0.05 test would be carried out for the primary endpoint.

Table 7.1 demonstrates the results of the trial on a primary endpoint and three secondary endpoints. Under the prospectively specified 0.05 rule, this trial has yielded a positive finding for the

Table 7.1. *P* values for Endpoints in
Concordantly Executed Clinical Trial

Endpoints	*P* Values
Primary Endpoint P1	0.040
Secondary Endpoint S1	0.070
Secondary Endpoint S2	0.010
Secondary Endpoint S3	0.001

primary endpoint. In addition, many workers would feel comfortable with the determination that S3 ($p = 0.001$) is positive and perhaps, would advocate that S2 ($p = 0.010$) is positive as well. These conclusions might even be supported by a rudimentary consideration of type I error. The line of reasoning might be that, if the endpoints (and the alpha accumulation) were considered in the order P1, S3, S2, and S1, accumulating type I error with each decision, the cumulative type I error for first P1 followed by S3 is less than 0.05, supporting the positive interpretation of S3. However, this non-prospective, data-based line of reasoning offers no protection from the consideration of other endpoint orderings equally admissible in this post hoc approach. For example, one could consider the endpoints (and accumulate alpha) in the order P1, S1, S2, S3. Beginning with P1, the accumulation of type I error for P1 and S1 is well above the 0.05 line, and neither endpoint S2 nor endpoint S3 could be considered positive. With no investigator-sponsored prospective statement, all endpoint orderings are worthy of consideration, and we have no guide on how to accumulate alpha. If one is not concerned with type I error accumulation, then S3 is positive. On the other hand, some consideration for the magnitude of type I error allocated (admittedly post hoc consideration) would lead to a negative S3 result (assuming adequate power S3 result).

In this example, the determination of endpoint significance requires focusing not just on the magnitude of the *p* values but also on the order in which one considers the secondary endpoints! This state of affairs is at best discomfiting.

The difficulty here is that, although there is not such great emphasis on secondary endpoints at a trial's inception, their findings receive important emphasis at the trial's conclusion. Thus the inclusion of secondary endpoints adds a new complexity to the interpretation of trial results. The "don't ask, don't tell" approach to the interpretation of these additional endpoints yields only bitter fruit. Who holds the responsibility to sort this out? The physician-scientists who designed the trial.

Community Expectations vs. Mandate Abrogation

We have seen that the thoughtless application of traditional rules, germane only for single-endpoint studies, to trials with multiple endpoints can lead to unfortunate complexities in clinical trial interpretation. Physician-scientists, the designers and executors of these large, collaborative efforts, are therefore obligated to design and execute their research programs to clarify rather than confuse the line of reasoning for the successful interpretation of all trial endpoints. They can fulfill this responsibility by first recalling their simultaneous responsibilities to protect both their individual patients ("first do no harm") and the community of patients to whom the experiments will be generalized. This responsibility requires the concordant execution of research programs that provide direct, clear type I and type II error interpretation. In order for physician-scientists to protect their patients from type I errors in these complicated multiple-endpoint trials, there must be explicit consideration of secondary endpoint findings. Since all medications have troublesome adverse effects, this community responsibility to reduce type I error is synonymous with reducing exposure of the patient community to noxious placebos. This responsibility also provides authority for investigators to set the alpha levels for each of the endpoints they intend to interpret—a mandate that requires the prospective delineation of their plan for alpha allocation. Fortunately, the investigators are in the best position to execute this mandate since, after all, they are often chosen for their scientific experience in general and their expertise in the use of the intervention medication in particular. The investigators use this experience to choose the study endpoints, ranking them with great deliberation as primary or secondary. This same knowledge places the investigators in the best possible position to choose alpha levels for each of the endpoints. By fulfilling their population protection responsibility prospectively and intelligently, the investigators have appropriately earned the opportunity to set the terms of the post trial debate on the importance of the experiment's findings.

However, in many trials the investigators abrogate this community responsibility. Investigators have become comfortable making statements concerning type I error (or at least, are comfortable with others making statements in their behalf) during the design phase of the trial; However, investigators often have difficulty-prospectively making statements about alpha allocation for secondary endpoints. They therefore provide tacit approval to the preeminence of a surprising finding which was not prospectively specified as primary, and surrender their authority for secondary endpoint interpretation to others.

Let the Investigators Decide After the Fact?

Of course the required prospective selection of alpha levels for secondary endpoints would be grimly met by some physician scientists, and rejected by others. Prospective alpha allocation requires the time consuming, careful and deliberate consideration of type I error rates for each and every prospectively identified endpoint. To many, this activity is tantamount to engaging in a pernicious abstraction; debates concerning alpha allocation for all of the trial's endpoints are seen as merely "jigging madly on the head of a pin." With the concept of a p value being entrenched, many of these investigators have come to the conclusion that reporting p values in the absence of alpha allocation is letting the data speak for itself. They believe that a new practice of drawing conclusions based on highly partitioned prospective type I error statements would blur the distinction between the experiment's objective scientific evidence and the investigators' intentions. After all, shouldn't the experimental conclusions reflect only the objective data and not the cleverness of the observer in "guessing the right alpha allocation" before the experiment is conducted? The driving theme is not "guessing the right alpha" but providing the right level of community protection.

Many investigators recoil from the notion of prospective alpha allocation for multiple endpoint trials. They argue that they should be required to present only the p values, with no prior statement about alpha allocation for secondary or perhaps even primary endpoints as well. In fact, p values are reported with no prior alpha allocation, the investigators contending that the experiment should be interpreted as positive if any endpoint is "significant at the 0.05 level" Reporting p values, they would suggest, presents an open display of the data, enabling readers to draw their own conclusions and "letting the data speak for themselves". My sad experience has been that those who argue that the data should "speak for themselves" are often the first ones to tell me what the data is saying. Authors may emphasize significant findings, perhaps not even reporting some non-significant endpoints [e.g., in the U. S. Carvedilol program]. Even if all endpoints are reported openly, authors and readers may still not appreciate the increased risk of a overall type I error rate. This point of view is, of course, understandable. These investigators most probably have never understood the sampling paradigm. They do not understand the alpha error concept, having impatiently but politely tolerated the brief discussion of alpha levels for the primary endpoint. They therefore will not sit still for detailed discussions of alpha allocation for additional endpoints. This may be a consequence of investigators who probably have not seriously reflected on their own important community protection responsibility. This responsibility requires both a clear understanding of and a tight rein on type I error rates. Letting investigators choose their own post hoc analysis plan ("let the data speak for themselves"), when there is not a prospective statement for alpha allocation is particularly worrisome. Not only is this alpha-corruptive, but the investigators will never shake themselves free of the suspicion that they chose the post hoc analyses that were most favorable to their case.

It is critical to understand that the scientific community's movement to the p value was not designed as a movement away from clear prospective statements about the significance test— only toward improved type I precision. The use of a p value was designed to refine the statement of "$p < 0.05$" to the sharper "$p = 0.025$." Therefore, the purpose of the p value was to sharpen the type I error estimate bound, not to reduce emphasis on prospective alpha control of the trial. P values were not developed as rationale for abandoning prospective thought for the trial outcomes. Community protection responsibilities require that investigators avoid the nominal p value as a determination of a finding of significance.

However, when the investigators fail the scientific community by not prospectively specifying the type I error strategy, post-experimental interpretations must be applied. Such post hoc strategies[10] are woefully inferior to a prospectively stated strategy by the investigators, since they are almost exclusively data driven. Another reason to disregard *post hoc* analyses is that commonly only a fraction of all possible analyses are presented. I think that a more reasonable path of analysis and alpha accumulation begins with the primary endpoint. Assess the statistical significance of the test statistic, then proceed through the secondary and tertiary prospectively stated endpoints, accumulating alpha until the maximum tolerable limit is achieved. Thus, if the maximum alpha allocated for the study is 0.05 and this type I error is exceeded for the primary endpoint, the p values for secondary endpoints cannot contribute to the argument of intervention benefit since the allocated alpha has been exceeded. This plan is inferior to a prospectively provided analysis plan by the investigators, and therefore should used only as a last resort.

Throwing the Baby Out with the Bath Water? Negative Trials with Positive Secondary Endpoints

The case of carvedilol was an example of a clinical trial which is negative for the primary endpoint but has positive findings either for secondary endpoints or in post hoc analyses. Interpreting such programs can be very frustrating, and this contentious setting has been the focus of sharp and spirited debate recently [1,2,5,6,7]. There is wisdom in the comments from Friedman et. al. [8] who state "it is more reasonable to calculate sample size based on one primary response variable comparison [i.e., emphasize the finding for the primary endpoint] and be cautious in claiming significant results for other comparisons." However, the degree to which investigators violate this principle in interpreting trial results sug-

---

[10] A *post hoc* strategy is a data analysis not prospectively stated in the protocol, motivated by the appearance of a finding in the data.

gests that this wisdom is not well appreciated. The price we seem to have paid for the profligate use of p values is a wholesale movement away from prospective declarations about all trial endpoints. Alpha allocation in trials with multiple endpoints and multiple treatment arms is more necessary than in experiments with one endpoint because of the alpha complexity. Wasteful interpretations of nominal p values discards this discipline when it is most needed.

Scientists who have invested time in a clinical trial, only to have it be negative for the primary endpoint too often throw all the caution of Friedman to the wind. In these circumstances, the primary endpoint, which had been chosen with great care and had been afforded particular attention during the trial, is unceremoniously unseated. Like the "crazy aunt in the attic," the negative primary endpoint receives little attention in the end, is referred to only obliquely or in passing, and is left to languish in scientific backwaters, as findings for positive endpoints (sometimes prospectively stated, sometimes not) are shoved to the forefront.

Some would argue that the conservative alpha allocation strategy advocated here throws out the "baby" of scientific progress with the "bath water" of alpha hypersensitivity [2]. Opinions on both the necessity and the strategy of alpha allocation are diverse [9–15]. These are contentious issues, but guidance for the selection of endpoints in clinical trials is available [9]. Scientists have developed multiple comparisons [16–17] and global hypothesis tests [18] to aid in the interpretation of clinical experiments with multiple treatment arms and multiple endpoints. The use of multiple comparison procedures based on the Bonferroni method [11] has invoke strong criticism from Rothman [15]. He states that such tools trivialize the possible hypothesis testing outcomes by reducing the maximum p value acceptable for a positive finding to a level that seems to preclude proclaiming any effect as positive. There are various strategies to interpret the family of p values from an experiment and various multiple comparison procedures available. However, because of either resultant alpha thresholds which are too low for investigators to accept, or comprehension difficulties for the nonstatisticians who must make policy decisions involving the experiment's results, these erudite solutions are often not invoked. Unfortunately, easily understood evolutions in p value interpretation have not kept pace with the increasing complexity of clinical research programs.

Conclusions

The two conflicting forces of endpoint abundance (the desire to measure many different clinical assessments at the end of an experiment) and interpretive parsimony (the alpha level and therefore the success of the trial rest on the interpretation of one and only one endpoint) bedevils investigators as they plan their experiments How can all of this information on nonprimary endpoints be interpreted when the medical and scientific community focus on the experimental p value for the primary endpoint of a trial? What is the correct interpretation of a trial that is negative for its primary endpoint, but has nominally statistically significant secondary endpoints? If a trial has two active arms and one placebo arm, must a single comparison take precedence?

These are difficult questions. The thesis of this introductory chapter is that it should no longer be sufficient to let investigators stand idly by, mute on the level of significance required for secondary endpoint determination. This policy is at best confusing and at worst exposes the community to harm through elevated type I error levels and its consequent exposure to noxious placebos. Investigators must wield their community protection mandate intelligently, sensitively, and effectively. The tack we will develop in the next chapter provides investigators the framework to choose the alpha levels in great detail a priori with the full freedom their community mandate provides.

References

1. Packer, M., Bristow, M.R. and Cohn, J.N. (1996) "The effect of carvedilol on morbidity and mortality in patients with chronic heart failure," New England Journal of Medicine 334:1349–1355.
2. Fisher, L., (1999) "Carvedilol and the FDA approval process: the FDA paradigm and reflections upon hypotheses testing," Controlled Clinical Trials 20:16–39.
3. Lewis, J.A. (1995) "Statistical Issues in the Regulation of Medicines," Statistics in Medicine 14:127–136.
4. Pocock, S.J., Geller, N.L., and Tsiatis, A.A., (1987) "The analysis of multiple endpoints in clinical trials," Biometrics 43:487–498.
5. Moyé, L.A., and Abernethy, D., (1996) "Carvedilol in Patients with Chronic Heart Failure," Letter New England Journal of Medicine 335:1318–1319.

6. Packer, M., Cohn, J.N., and Colucci, W.S. "Response to Moyé and Abernethy," *New England Journal of Medicine* 335:1318–1319.

7. Moyé, L.A., (1999) "*P* Value Interpretation in Clinical Trials. The Case for Discipline," *Controlled Clinical Trials* 20:40–49.

8. Friedman, L., Furberg, C., and DeMets, D., (1996) *Fundamentals of Clinical Trials*, Third Edition, Mosby. Meinert, C.L., (1986) *Clinical Trials Design, Conduct, and Analysis*, Oxford University Press, New York.

9. Dowdy, S., Wearden, S., (1991) *Statistics for Research*, Second Edition, John Wiley and Sons, New York.

10. Dubey, S.D. "Adjustment of p values for multiplicities of inter-connecting symptoms" in *Statistics in the pharmaceutical industry* Second Edition. Buncher, R.C. and Tsay, J.Y. Editors, Marcel Dekker Inc., New York.

11. Snedecor, G.W., Cochran, W.G., (1980), *Statistical Methods* Seventh Edition, Iowa State University Press, Iowa.

12. Gnosh, B.K., Sen, P.K. *Handbook of Sequential Analysis*, Marcel Dekker Inc., New York.

13. Miller, R.G., (1981) *Simultaneous Statistical Inference* Second Edition, Springer-Verlag, New York.

14. Anderson, T.W., (1984) *An Introduction to Multivariate Statistical Analysis* Second Edition, John Wiley and Sons, New York.

15. Rothman, R.J., (1990) "No adjustments are needed for multiple comparisons," *Epidemiology* 1:43–46.

16. Simes, R.J., (1986) "An improved Bonferonni procedure for multiple tests of significance," *Biometrika* 73:751–754.

17. Worsley, K.L (1982) "An improved Bonferroni inequality and applications," *Biometrika* 69:297–302.

18. Pocock, S.J., Geller, N.L., and Tsiasis, A.A., (1987) "The analysis of multiple endpoints in clinical trials," *Biometrics* 423:487–498.

P values and Multiple Endpoints II: Noxious Placebos in the Population

8

CHAPTER

Noxious Placebo Protection

The previous chapter motivated complicated work. Because it has the advantage of fiscal efficiency and buttreses a causality argument, the clinical trial with multiple treatment arms and/or multiple endpoints is here to stay. It is the physician-scientist's responsibility to incorporate these dual concerns of efficiency and epidemiology within the paradigm of significance testing. The investigator's community protection responsibilities clearly require the unambiguous interpretation of type I errors in multiple endpoint clinical experiments. The *p* value is the probability that the therapy efficacy contained in the sample, through the play of chance, does not reflect the truth of no efficacy in the population. The occurrence of this (type I) error leads to the community of patients being exposed to a medication which is not effective but produces side effects. Thus, we may view a *p* value in therapy trials as the probability that a noxious or poison placebo is deemed (through the play of chance) to be effective. This noxious placebo may spread through the community as the false result is picked up and disseminated through the printed and visual media, as well as through regulatory channel of the F. D. A. Thus, in a concordantly executed experiment, the smaller the *p* value, the smaller the probability that a noxious placebo will be deemed effective.

In this setting with multiple significance testing, the community has a greater risk (through a greater type I error) of being exposed to a medication that is deemed "safe," yet produce real harm through side effects. Sometimes the side effects can be very serious. If the medication is not effective and the investigator concludes that it is effective, the population exposed to the medication will receive no efficacy, but real harm. This risk must be minimized to provide adequate safeguards for community health, to insure that patients receive not just risk, but benefit from the intervention. This interpretation requires that the total type I error of the experiment should be prospectively conserved.

The concept presented here is an adaptation of multiple testing, taking advantage of the embedded opportunity prospective designs afford to allocate alpha at different levels for different endpoints. This development will proceed slowly, starting with alpha allocation strategy from the simplest of problems, adding layer upon layer of complexity to the apportionment of alpha in clinical experiments with multiple endpoints. At the conclusion of this chapter, it is hoped that the reader will be adept at going through the steps of apportioning alpha intelligently, sensitively, asymmetrically, and ethically to clinical trials with multiple endpoints and treatment arms.

PA³S — The Prospective Asymmetric Alpha Allocation System

Research investigators can begin the process of alpha conservation by choosing all endpoints prospectively. Thus they will appropriately set the standard by which the experiment will be judged. However, they can further strengthen their experimental design by choosing the allocation of the type I error. Alpha should be allocated to protocol-specified hypotheses and protocol-specified subgroup analyses. Our purpose here is to advance the notion of a prospective asymmetric alpha allocation system (PA³S—pronounced "P-A-three-System"), introducing trial result descriptions in terms of trial endpoints. The combination of a prospective allocation argument and new terminology provides the setting in which an experiment that did not reject the null hypothesis for the primary endpoint but does reject the null hypothesis for secondary endpoints may be considered positive as described the previous chapter. In addition, we will make an argument for differentiating between the type I error of the experiment (experimental alpha α_E) and the total type I error for the primary endpoint, α_P. We will demonstrate that an intelligently considered increase in experimental alpha above the level of 0.05 serves the useful purposes of conserving sample size and preserving consistency with past standards of strength of evidence for the primary endpoint of clinical trials.

The prospective alpha allocation scheme is an adaptation of the simple Bonferroni procedure[1] [1,2]. We will begin with a simple alpha computation. Define experimental (or trial) alpha α_E, as the total type I error in the experiment. As the total alpha alloted in this experiment will be for each of the primary and secondary endpoints. Each will have alpha assigned prospectively, α_P for the primary endpoint and α_S for the secondary endpoint. Since one of the goals of the investigator is to set an upper bound for the experimental type I error, there are limitations placed on α_P and α_S. We begin by writing the probability of no type I error in the experiment as the product of the probability of no type I error on the primary endpoint and the probability no type I error on the secondary endpoint.

$$1 - \alpha_E = (1 - \alpha_P)(1 - \alpha_S) \tag{8.1}$$

and easily find that

$$\alpha_E = 1 - (1 - \alpha_P)(1 - \alpha_S) \tag{8.2}$$

The probability invoked here is that of the event "at least one alpha error", described in Snedecor and Cochran[1], page 116.[1] Thus, α_E is the probability of making at least one type I error i.e., an error on either the primary endpoint, the secondary endpoint, or both. This formula readily generalizes to the experiment which has n_p primary endpoints and n_s secondary endpoints.

---

[1] This assumes independence between the type I error event for the primary endpoint and the type I error event for the secondary endpoint. Relaxing this assumption requires specific information about the nature of the dependence between primary and secondary endpoints, which will be trial specific. A case of dependency will be presented later in this chapter.

$$\alpha_E = 1 - \left[\prod_{i=1}^{n_p}(1 - \alpha_{p,i})\right]\left[\prod_{j=1}^{n_s}(1 - \alpha_{s,j})\right] \qquad (8.3)$$

From this one equation,[2] the cumulative total alpha expended in the experiment, α_E, can be computed from the α_{pi}'s and the $\alpha_{s,i}$'s. Also, if we are given an initial value of α_E and each of the $\alpha_{p,i}$'s, we can compute the values of $\alpha_{s,i}$'s. We can therefore easily compute the total alpha, given the alpha levels chosen for the primary and secondary endpoints, as well as compute the alpha levels for the secondary endpoints, given the total alpha for the experiment and the alpha levels for the primary endpoint(s). The simple key to PA^{3}S, is to choose the type I error levels for each of the endpoints separately, then use equation (2) to compute the total alpha expended. I provide several intuitive examples with simple computations to motivate this function's use. We will assume that all hypothesis testing is two-tailed (symmetric) initially[3], and relax the symmetry assumption later in this chapter.

Scenario 1.
Consider an experiment that will randomize patients to one of two treatment arms to an intervention designed to treat congestive heart failure. The primary endpoint for the trial is total mortality. The three secondary endpoints are hospitalization for heart failure, progression of heart failure, and exercise tolerance. The investigators believe that the state of treatment for congestive heart failure is stable and well accepted, with known side effect profiles, and that physicians in general believe the benefits of these medications are worth the risk. Therefore, the scientific and patient communities require strong evidence of benefit before this new therapy to be with its own, new side effect profile, is introduced. In this situation, it would be dangerous to conclude from the trial that the medication is effective if it is not since it would unleash on congestive heart failure patients in the community an ineffective compound that will do harm through its side effects. Therefore, we can tolerate only a small probability that a population noxious placebo is demonstrating sample efficacy. This is the type I error the investigator wishes to minimize.

Although the investigator places priority on the primary end-

---

[2] This probability has its upper bound approximated by Bonferroni's inequality, but an exact treatment will be developed here.
[3] The disadvantages of symmetry are pointed out in chapter 6.

Table 8.1. Alpha Allocation : $\alpha_E = 0.05$ (two sided)

Endpoint	Allocated Alpha
Primary Endpoint	0.02000
Total Mortality	0.02000
Secondary Endpoints	0.03061
Hospitalization for CHF	0.01031
Progression of CHF	0.01031
Exercise Tolerance	0.01031

point of total mortality, he would like to carry out a significance test on each of the secondary endpoints which are of equal concern for the propagation of type I error and will be assigned the same alpha levels. He sets $\alpha_E = 0.05$ and chooses $\alpha_P = 0.02$. From these choices, we easily compute the available alpha for the secondary endpoints from equation 8.1 as

$$\alpha_S = 1 - \frac{1 - \alpha_E}{1 - \alpha_p} = 1 - \frac{(0.95)}{(0.98)} = 0.03061$$

So $\alpha_S = 0.03061$ is the available type I error for the family of secondary endpoints. Apportioning this equally among the three endpoints, we find

$$1 - 0.03061 = (1 - \alpha_S)^3$$

and $\alpha_S = 0.01031$. An alpha allocation table assembled by the investigators and supplied prospectively in the experiment's protocol (Table 8.1) is an unambiguous statement of the investigators' plans for assessing the impact of the experimental intervention.

The Bonferroni procedure, as it is usually applied, would have apportioned alpha equally across the primary and secondary endpoints. However, in this particular example, the investigator exercised his authority to distinguish between the alpha levels for the primary endpoint and the alpha levels for the secondary endpoints. Once he determined the alpha level available for the secondary endpoints, he allocated alpha equally across the secondary level[4].

---

[4] Note that the total allocated alpha errors for the secondary endpoint is not the sum of the alpha allocated for each of the secondary endpoints. Similarly $\alpha_E \neq \alpha_P + \alpha_S$. This is a predictable and essentially harmless comsequence of applying equation (8.3).

Table 8.2.   Alpha Allocation : $\alpha_E = 0.05$ (two-sided)

Endpoint	Allocated Alpha
A_1 vs. Placebo Comparison	**0.02532**
Primary Endpoint	
Total Mortality	0.02000
Secondary Endpoints	0.00543
Intermittent Claudication	0.00272
Unstable Angina	0.00272
A_2 vs. Placebo Comparison	**0.02532**
Primary Endpoint	
Total Mortality	0.02000
Secondary Endpoints	0.00543
Intermittent Claudication	0.00272
Unstable Angina	0.00272

Scenario 2

An investigator is designing a clinical trial with a placebo and two treatment arms A_1 and A_2. There is equal interest is testing 1) A_1 against placebo and 2) A_2 against placebo. For each of these tests, there is one primary endpoint, total mortality, and two secondary endpoints (intermittent claudication and unstable angina). The investigator sets the total alpha for the experiment, $\alpha_E = 0.05$, to be divided equally between the two tests (A_1 vs. placebo and A_2 vs. placebo). We find

$$1 - \alpha_E = (1 - \alpha_{A_1})(1 - \alpha_{A_2}) = (1 - \alpha_A)^2.$$

revealing

$$\alpha_{A_1} = \alpha_{A_2} = 1 - (1 - \alpha_E)^{0.5} = 0.02532.$$

Thus 0.02532 is available for comparison of each of the treatment arms to the placebo arm of the experiment. Consider comparing treatment arm A_1 against placebo. The investigator allows 0.02 of this for the primary endpoint comparison of A_1 against placebo. He then computes the remaining alpha to be allotted, distributing this equally across the two secondary endpoints. The investigator computes

$$\alpha_S^* = 1 - \left(\frac{1 - 0.02532}{1 - 0.02}\right)^{0.5} = 0.00272$$

Since A_2 would be handled analogously, the allocation of alpha for the endpoints can be completed (Table 8.2)

Table 8.3.   Alpha Allocation : $\alpha_E = 0.05$ (two sided)

Endpoint	Alpha Allocated (Design)	P Value (Execution)
Primary Endpoint	0.02500	
Total Mortality	0.02500	0.00100
Secondary Endpoints	0.02564	
Hospitalization for CHF	0.01290	0.02000
Progression of CHF (medication status)	0.01290	0.00400

Note here that the investigator could have different levels of alpha for the system of tests for treatment A_1 and the system involving A_2 vs. placebo.

Scenario 3

Consider a two armed trial testing the impact of an intervention to treat congestive heart failure (CHF) on a primary endpoint of total mortality and each of two secondary endpoints, hospitalization for CHF and CHF progression. The investigators set alpha, $\alpha_E = 0.05$, and assign 0.025 for the primary endpoint, providing each of these secondary endpoints equal weight. Applying equation 1, the investigators compute an alpha allocation table (Table 8.3).

Let's turn to the execution of the experiment. Assume the experiment is concordantly executed,[5] and the significance of the endpoints assessed. The p value for the primary endpoint is less than that allocated, and the finding for the primary endpoint is positive. The overall alpha expended in the experiment is

$$= 1 - (1 - 0.00100)(1 - 0.02000)(1 - 0.00400) = 0.02490$$

much less than the 0.05 allocated. However, the findings for hospitalization for CHF did not reach the threshold of significance prospectively allocated for this experiment so the findings for that endpoint should be interpreted as negative. Some workers, focused on the 0.02 p value of the hospitalization for CHF endpoint, would have difficulty with this conclusion. However, the investigators,

---

[5] Without concordant execution (see Chapter 2), the p values from this experiment would be meaningless, even with superb prospective alpha allocation. Discordant experiments (which allow the data to alter the analysis plan of the experiment) will undo intelligently and prospectively chosen alpha allocation schemes.

having set alpha prospectively have the authority to provide the first, best assessment of the findings of this experiment.

Some Interim Comments on PA³S

PA³S allows investigators to select α_E and the level of alpha errors for each of the primary and secondary endpoints prior to the experiment, providing a framework by which they can translate their mandate for community protection from type I errors into a thoughtful consideration of the alpha error appropriate for each endpoint. Since the PA³S is prospectively applied, it should only be used for prospectively determined endpoints (i.e., formal hypothesis testing), and not for the less formal exploratory analyses designed to identify relationships not anticipated at the experiment's inception.[6] I would recommend that, at the trial's inception, a PA³S table be constructed, be made part of the experiment's protocol, and be disseminated to the scientific community. Upon the experiment's conclusion, the *p* value[7] column is completed and the finished table is distributed with the study results.

It would be useful to examine several possible conclusions of experiments executed under the PA³S framework. Consider a clinical trial investigating the effect of a single intervention to reduce morbidity and mortality in a population of patients with congestive heart failure. There is a control arm and a treatment arm. The primary endpoint of the experiment is total mortality, but there is strong interest in examining the effect of therapy on changes in left ventricular ejection fraction (secondary endpoint S1), worsening heart failure (secondary endpoint S2), and total hospitalizations for heart failure (secondary endpoint S3). Using the above scheme, the investigators choose to allocate 0.05 alpha (i.e., set $\alpha = 0.05$), distributing it among the primary and secondary endpoints. The investigators allocate 0.035 of the total alpha to the primary endpoint, distributing the remaining 0.015 alpha equally among the secondary endpoints. This distribution insures that the total type I error for the trial is 0.05, meeting the investigators obligation for community protection from type I error.

---

[6] Exploratory analysis and its implications are discussed in chapter 11.
[7] Alpha is the description of type I error allocation prior to the experiment, and p value is the measured type I error as a result of the experiment.

Table 8.4. Sample Results—Alpha Allocation and Three Scenarios

	Alpha Allocation	Scenario 1 Alpha Expenditure	Scenario 2 Alpha Expenditure	Scenario 3 Alpha Expenditure
Total	0.050			
Primary Endpoints	0.035	0.020	0.040	0.080
Secondary Endpoint	0.015			
S1	0.005	0.070	0.070	0.070
S2	0.005	0.080	0.010	0.010
S3	0.005	0.100	0.001	0.001

We may examine some interesting implications of this alpha allocation decision by considering three different clinical scenarios, each reflecting a hypothetical experimental result (Table 8.4). Assume that each experiment is concordantly executed, and the hypothesis test for each endpoint in each scenario is adequately powered.[8] In scenario 1, the experiment produced a p value 0.020 for total mortality. In the customary manner of interpreting clinical trials, this finding would be considered a positive result. This is true under PA³S as well, since 0.020 is less than the alpha prospectively allocated for the primary endpoint. Consideration of the large p values for each of the secondary endpoints S1, S2, and S3 supports the conclusion that the study is negative[9] for all secondary endpoints, although the experiment as a whole would most assuredly be interpreted as positive based on the finding for the primary endpoint by either the customary procedure or PA³S.

The circumstances are different in scenario 2. Under the customary 0.05 rule, scenario 2 has yielded a positive finding for the primary endpoint. In addition, many workers would feel comfortable with the determination that S3 is positive $(p = 0.001)$, and perhaps, would advocate that S2 is positive $(p = 0.010)$ as well. This is the example developed in chapter 7, in which the conclusion was order dependent. However, a prospective alpha allocation scheme would lead to order independent, unambiguous results. The p value of the primary endpoint (0.040) exceeds the alpha allocated for it and thus would be interpreted as negative under PA³S. In addition, the small p value for endpoint S3 (0.001)

---

[8] The concept of power is discussed in chapter 5.
[9] The conclusion that the study is negative assumes the study is adequately powered.

would allow a positive conclusion for S3 since it is less than the 0.005 allocated to it. Thus the study would be interpreted under PA^{3}S as positive, even though the primary endpoint finding was negative. Note that the conclusion from both the PA^{3}S and customary procedures for *p* value interpretation is that the study is positive, albeit for different reasons. It would be usefully to distinguish between these modes of positivity.

Scenario 3 represents a common experimental motif and is of great concern. Here, the *p* value for the primary endpoint is greater than the allocated alpha and would be interpreted as negative (again, assuming adequate power). This is also the conclusion of the customary 0.05 rule for the primary endpoint. The experiment is negative and, customarily to the chagrin of the investigators, this is where the interpretation ends, since many workers reject the notion of a positive trial with a negative primary endpoint. In this view, the primary endpoint of the trial is considered supreme; all alpha is expended on the primary endpoint and the conclusion of this single hypothesis test determines whether the trial is a success or a failure. With no prospective alpha allocation scheme, the common conclusion would be that scenario 3 was negative (again assuming adequate power). However, use of the PA^{3}S admits an additional possibility. Scenario 3 would be considered a positive result even in the absence of a primary endpoint *p* value less than the allocated alpha, because the *p* value for the secondary endpoint S3 was less than the a priori defined alpha allocation. The prospective alpha allocation scheme admits the possibility of a positive trial with a negative primary endpoint finding, while at the same time conserving type I error.

Scenario 2 and scenario 3 suggest that we develop a more useful definition of a positive trial. In the past, experiments were considered positive if and only if the *p* value for the primary endpoint was less than the alpha allocated to it (most commonly, 0.05). Decisions about secondary endpoints have always been murky in this circumstance when the p value for the secondary endpoint was less than the traditional 0.05 value. However, we might more constructively (and more objectively) view a positive experiment as one in which any prospectively defined endpoint's *p* value is less than its prospectively allocated alpha level. However, in describing results, it would be helpful to unambiguously distinguish between a clinical trial that was positive for the primary endpoint and one that was deemed positive based on secondary endpoint findings.

Notation

In both scenario 2 and scenario 3 a trial with negative finding for the primary endpoint but a positive finding for a secondary endpoint is considered positive under PA^{3}S. If trial results as represented by these two scenarios are to be accepted as positive, it would be helpful to have notation and nomenclature to differentiate these types of results from other trial results more traditionally deemed positive. That nomenclature is easily developed here.

Consider a clinical trial with exactly one primary endpoint and exactly one secondary endpoint. For each of these two endpoints, a hypothesis test is executed and interpreted, and for each endpoint, we will conclude that the test is either positive (the p value from the hypothesis test is less than the allocated alpha), negative (the p value from the hypothesis test is greater than the allocated alpha, and the test was adequately powered) or inconclusive (the p value from the hypothesis test is greater than the allocated alpha, but the test had insufficient power). We shall describe the findings of such a clinical trial as $P_a S_b$ where the subscript a denotes the conclusion from the primary hypothesis test, and the subscript b denotes the conclusion from the hypothesis test of the secondary endpoint. The values of each of a and b can be p(positive), n(negative) or i(inconclusive). With this notation, a clinical trial which is positive for the primary endpoint and positive for the secondary endpoint would be denoted as $P_p S_p$. Analogously, a trial in which each of the endpoints were found to be negative is a $P_n S_n$ trial. A $P_p S_I$ trial has a positive primary endpoint and an inconclusive finding for the secondary endpoint due to inadequate power.

Of course, clinical trials often have more than one secondary endpoint and sometimes have more than one primary endpoint. We can embed this multiplicity of findings for these multiple endpoints into this notation by stipulating P_p if at least one of the primary endpoints is positive and P_n if all of the primary endpoints in the trial are negative. Denote the finding that some of the primary endpoints are negative and the remaining ones uninformative as P_{ni}. For example, a trial with one negative and one positive primary endpoint, and secondary endpoints, one negative and one inconclusive, would be denoted as a $P_p S_{ni}$ trial.

No investigator (myself included) can resist the opportunity to use a dataset to address questions that were not prospectively stated. Often, a new advance may suggest a question that the investigators did not know to ask at the trial's inception. For an example, investigators might draw blood from patients at baseline and store the blood for future analyses, which cannot yet be described because the necessary technology although anticipated, is not yet available. In addition, journal editors and reviewers sometimes ask for additional, nonprospectively identified analyses to support a reviewed manuscript's thesis. We may include the conclusions of such hypothesis-generating endeavors by adding an H_c at the end of the trial designation. Thus, a trial which is negative for all of the primary endpoints, negative or uninformative on secondary endpoints, and positive for some hypothesis generating effort would be designated $P_n S_{ni} H_p$.

An advantage of this classification is that the notation differentiates trials that are positive for the primary endpoint from trials that are negative for the primary endpoint but positive for secondary endpoints. We can now specifically and concisely contrast the impact of PA^{3}S application with the traditional approach. With no prior alpha allocation, a $P_n S_p$ trial would not be considered positive. This is because, in the absence of a prospective statement by the investigators, a reasonable path of analysis and alpha accumulation begins with the primary endpoint, assessing its statistical significance, then proceeding through the secondary and tertiary prospectively stated endpoints, accumulating alpha until the maximum tolerable limit is achieved. Thus, if the maximum alpha allocated for the study is 0.05 and this type I error is exceeded for the primary endpoint, the p values for secondary endpoints cannot contribute to the argument of intervention benefit so the $P_n S_p$ study be considered negative. However, as we have seen from scenarios 2 and 3, the prospective alpha allocation can produce a $P_n S_p$ result which should be considered a positive trial, since the positive findings for the secondary endpoint occur without exceeding the α_E cap. As long as alpha allocation is provided prospectively, the $P_n S_p$ experiment deserves no pejorative appellation and should not be considered a second-class result. This represents a fundamental change in the interpretation of clinical trials.

Examples of the use of this notation (the alpha allocation is admittedly applied *post hoc*) appear in Table 8.5. For example, in the Survival and Ventricular Enlargement (SAVE) trial, the results were positive for the primary endpoint of total mortality. The secondary endpoints of the trial included hospitalization for heart

Table 8.5. Classification of a Selection of Clinical Trials by Endpoint Findings

Clinical Trial	Findings	Classifi- cation n
SAVE—Survival and Ventricular Enlargement [3]	PEP: Positive for total mortality SEP: Positive for hospitalization for CHF Positive for worsening CHF Negative for protocol defined myocardial infarction	P_pS_p
CARE—Cholesterol and Recurrent Events [4]	PEP: Positive for CHD death/MI SEP: Positive for revascularization Positive for stroke	P_pS_p
SHEP—Systolic Hypertension in the Elderly [5]	PEP: Positive for fatal and nonfatal stroke SEP: Positive for myocardial infarction Positive for revascularization Positive for congestive heart failure	P_pS_p
NitroDur [6]—Post infarction nitrate paste use	PEP: Positive for change in end systolic volume ESVI SEP: Negative for post trial change in ESVI	P_pS_n
CAST [7]	PEP: Positive for harm for total mortality SEP: Positive for harm for cardiac mortality	$P^*_pS^*_p$
LRC(Lipid Research Clinics) [8]	PEP: Negative for reduction in CHD death/ myocardial infarction SEP: Positive	P_nS_p
Linet et. al. Magnetic Fields [9][10]	PEP: Negative for association between magnetic field proximity and acute lymphoblastic leukemia matched analysis SEP Negative for association between magnetic field proximity and acute lymphoblastic leukemia unmatched analysis	P_nS_n
Hayes, et. Al [10] Cardiac Function and Pacemakers	PEP: Negative for pacemaker disruption with normal cell phone use SEP: Positive for pacemaker disruption with unusual cell phone position	P_nS_p

* PEP denotes primary endpoint. SEP denotes secondary endpoint

[10] The Linet and Hayes studies both have the problem of non random assignment of exposure. As pointed out in chapter 3, the attribution of an effect to an exposure can be problematic in circumstances where there is no random exposure allocation.

failure, worsening heart failure, recurrent myocardial infarction, and deterioration in ejection fraction. Since several of these secondary endpoints were positive, the designation would be SAVE-P_pS_p. An asterisk is used to identify a harmful effect (e.g. CAST-$P^*{}_pS^*{}_p$)

The Sample Size Straightjacket

One difficulty in the implementation of PA^3S is the use of α_P as input to the sample size computation. The smaller the alpha error, the larger the sample size required to test the effect at that lower level of significance. If $\alpha_E = 0.05$ and $\alpha_P < \alpha_E$, the sample size based on this smaller α_P will be larger. Consider an experiment designed to detect the effect of an intervention on a primary endpoint of total mortality and a secondary endpoint of total hospitalizations. The investigators intend to compute the sample size of the trial based on the primary endpoint, planning to achieve a 20 percent reduction in total mortality from a control group total mortality rate of 15 percent with 80 percent power. The standard procedure would be to compute the sample size based on a formula such as

$$N = \frac{2[p_1(1 - p_1) + p_2(1 - p_2)][Z_{1-\alpha/2} - Z_\beta]^2}{[p_1 - p_2]^2} \qquad (8.4)$$

where N is the number of patients randomized to the placebo group plus the number of patients randomized to the active group, α = type I error, β = type II error, Z_c = the cth percentile from the standard normal probability distribution, p_1 = cumulative total mortality rate in the placebo group and p_2 = hypothesized total mortality rate in the active group[11]. In this case, $p_1 = 0.15$, $p_2 = 0.12$, $\alpha = 0.05$ and N is 4,060 for a type I error of 0.05.

However, using PA^3S, the investigators generate Table 8.6.

In this setting, although $\alpha_E = 0.05$, $\alpha_P = 0.03$. The sample size from formula (2) based on α_p is 4,699, and increase from the original sample size of 4,060. Furthermore, the increase in sample size does not insure adequate power for the secondary endpoints. Although this 16 percent increase in sample size is the price the

---

[11] Chapter 5 discusses sample size issues.

Table 8.6. Prospective Alpha Allocation for Sample Size Comparison

	Alpha Allocation	
Total	0.050	
Alpha for Primary Endpoint—Total Mortality	0.030	
Alpha for Secondary Endpoints—Total Hospitalizations	0.021	
S1		0.007
S2		0.007
S3		0.007

Table 8.7. Prospective Alpha Allocation for Sample Size Comparison

	Alpha Allocation	
Total	0.100	
Alpha for Primary Endpoint	0.050	
Alpha for Secondary Endpoints	0.053	
S1		0.018
S2		0.018
S3		0.018

investigators must pay to provide the possibility of a positive finding on the secondary endpoint (earning the right to claim not just P_pS_p positivity but P_nS_p positivity), the sample size increase is substantial and the added financial and logistical burden is worrisome.

Our discussion in chapter 2 grants the investigators the authority to be flexible in providing upper bounds on prospectively specified type I error levels. There we established that the investigators have earned the mandate to allocate alpha at other than the 0.05 level of significance. Although laudable, the scientific community and regulatory agencies would most likely raise concerns about this vitiation of the scientific evidence strength. The investigators could persuasively respond that the α_E they are accustomed to spending on the primary endpoint must now be shared over primary and secondary endpoints. A compromise would be to allow an increase in α_E to 0.10, but to cap α_P at 0.05. Thus, the investigators would be free to construct an alpha allocation as in Table 8.7.

In this case, α_P is retained at 0.05, permitting adequate power for the primary endpoint with the original sample size of 4,066. This recommendation permits the primary endpoint to be maintained at the 0.05 level of statistical significance, but the prospective alpha specification (0.053) is more lenient for the secondary endpoints, due to the increase in α_E from 0.05 to 0.10. The increase in $\forall_E$ has permitted consistency in strength of evidence for the primary endpoint, expressed concern for the sample size, and still allowed ample possibility for a P_nS_p positive trial. Some may argue that the threshold for a positive trial has been reduced by this strategy. However, in the PA³S framework, a positive trial is one in which the p value for the prospectively delineated endpoint is less than the maximum alpha level permitted. In current practice, there is no consistent, satisfactory framework in which to consider P_nS_p positivity.

By enforcing experimental concordance, the investigators ease the task of interpreting their research. However, rigor and discipline in experimental execution should not exclude the prospective determination of acceptable alpha error levels. This is a serious investigator obligation, since both population and patient protection are the responsibility of clinical scientists. Capping α_P provides both some protection for the scientific community and relief for the investigators. It also is a starting point for breaking the 0.05 stranglehold on investigators. Although there is no theoretical justification for α_P of 0.05, it cannot be denied that the history of clinical trial significance thresholds nevertheless exerts considerable influence. Considering experiments with $\alpha_P > 0.05$ as positive would be seen by many as inconsistent with previous work and weaken the strength of evidence standard. It may be difficult to integrate the findings from these experiments (considered by some to be diluted) into the scientific fund of knowledge. Keeping α_P fixed at 0.05 maintains some consistency with the past, although as discussed in chapter three, the investigators have earned the right to relax the standard. In addition, since sample sizes are computed based on α_P, maintaining its level at 0.05 does not lead to sample size increases. Thus, investigators pay no penalty in sample size by using PA³S. By letting $\alpha_P = 0.05 < \alpha_E$, the sample size straightjacket that confined investigators even further in experimental design has been relieved. This would not be the case if α_E were set at 0.05, and $\alpha_P < \alpha_E$.

One might successfully argue that the admittedly conservative alpha allocation strategy is an inappropriate standard in the academic setting, where findings from secondary endpoints in pilot studies might be used to generate hypotheses for subsequent experiments. There are important criticisms of the analysis path approach which I advocate. However, it has the advantage of being disciplined, prospectively identified, and unambiguous in its interpretation. In rendering final judgment, we must therefore keep in mind what is best for the population at large, which often must bear the brunt of type I errors. The alpha allocation approach advocated here has the virtue of being prospectively defined, quantitative, and easy to reproduce. However, it must be noted that this procedure also has the weaknesses of its virtues. Because it is quantitative — it is also formal and restrictive. Because it is prospectively defined, it is also non-reactive to new information made available while the trial is in progress. An alternative approach would incorporate prior information about the relatively likelihood of the research effort's ability to produce a positive finding, and also develop a loss function for drawing the incorrect conclusion. Bayes procedures,[12] which incorporate the parameterization of prior information concerning an action and information from the experiment itself into a posterior decision rule using a credible region, have become of greater interest [24]. Much of clinical decision making is based on more than a single research program, and interpretation and subsequent actions are generally in the context of other information and other research, not solely based on a solitary p value. Therefore, the Bayesian approach would offer researchers a way to more accurately describe their own methods of implicitly integrating prior information into the consideration of the data at hand.

As we have pointed out earlier, many workers will be uncomfortable with the notion of prospective alpha allocation, believing that such an approach rewards only the clever alpha allocation guessers. What are the practical consequences of this concern? Consider the following hypothetical experiment in which two investigators each reasonably allocate alpha for a clinical trial involving primary and secondary endpoints as in Table 8.8

Each investigator has 0.100 alpha to allocate, and each chooses to allocate it differently. The first investigator places 0.05 on the one primary endpoint, and distributes the remaining 0.053 alpha among the secondary endpoints. The second investigator places less alpha on the primary endpoint, demonstrating increased in-

---

[12] The Bayes approach to significance testing is discussed in chapter 10.

Table 8.8. Hypothetical Alpha Allocation—Two Investigators

Endpoint	Investigator 1 Alpha Allocation		Investigator 2 Alpha Allocation		Actual Results	
Total Alpha	0.100		0.100			
Primary	0.050		0.030		0.040	
Secondary	0.053		0.072		0.053	
S1		0.018		0.040		0.030
S2		0.018		0.017		0.040
S3		0.018		0.017		0.040

terest in the secondary endpoints. When the actual results are reported, it seems at first glance that the investigators report the results differently. Investigator 1 would report the results as positive for the primary endpoint and negative for all secondary endpoints (P_pS_n). Investigator 2 reports a negative finding for the primary, but a positive finding for the secondary endpoint (P_nS_p). However, because of the prospective statement for alpha, each investigator is justified in calling the experiment positive. It is my view that reasonable alpha allocations produced from careful thought applied to the intervention-endpoint relationship will lead to coherent interpretations of the dataset. Small differences in prior alpha allocation can lead to differences in the interpretation of a particular endpoint but are unlikely to lead to differences in the global interpretation of the experiment with a well chosen cadre of primary/secondary endpoints. However, each allocation should have a justification that is based on a consensus of other investigators and reviewers.

The successful utilization of the P_aS_b system must incorporate the issue of power. When rejection of the null hypothesis is not possible, the conclusion is based on the power. If the power is high, the result of the hypothesis test is negative. If the power is low, the "conclusion" is only that the hypothesis test was uninformative or inconclusive. This is true for any prospectively stated endpoint. Of course, difficulty arises for secondary endpoints. Primary endpoints should always have adequate power but it is difficult to insure adequate power for secondary endpoints. For example, the primary endpoint of a trial to test a randomly assigned intervention to reduce ischemic heart disease may be a combination of fatal myocardial infarction and survival but nonfatal myocardial infarction. A reasonable secondary endpoint could be fatal myocardial infarction. However, the necessity of trial cost-effectiveness often provides only the bare minimum of power (e.g., 80 percent) for the combined primary endpoint, insuring the power for the fatal myocardial infarction endpoint with its lower cumulative incidence rate, will be lower (for the same type I error rate and the same efficacy). Thus deciding whether the value of b in P_aS_b is n or i depends on the power of the secondary endpoint hypothesis test.

The development here subsumes the possibility of correlation between endpoints. Dependency of endpoints leads to a different computation of alpha allocation then in equation 8.1, and, when there is dependency in the endpoints 8.1 can be much too conservative [19]. In addition, the work of Westfall and Young [11] has demonstrated that corrections for multiple testing can be made accurately through either permutation type or bootstrapping type resampling. These approaches offer substantial improvements over the usual Bonferroni type of adjustments because the dependence structures and other useful distributional characteristics are automatically incorporated into the analysis. There are other acceptable approaches as well. The use of a rank ordering strategy for endpoints is an important consideration, and can be useful in a hierarchy of events. However the utility of these approaches vastly improved with a clear prospective statement from the investigators, including the precise decision path they intend to follow in the post trial analysis. This strategy also allows for an unambiguous interpretation of p values and can fully incorporate the concept that $\alpha_p < \alpha_E$. In addition, a useful Bayesian approach to this issue has been addressed Wesfall, et. al. [16], and the notion of posterior probabilities as a replacement for p values remains attractive. However, the thrust of our argument remains unchanged. There are several admissible ways of allocating alpha. One of them (based on an assessment of endpoint dependency) should be used.

This discussion does not explicitly consider alpha spending function during interim monitoring. This important concept can be incorporated by using the determinations from the allocation column of the PA^{3}S table as input to the alpha spending function approaches, using either sequential boundary procedures [12–13] or those of conditional power procedures [14–15].

An Ethical Move to Asymmetry

The preceding computations exemplify the prospective apportionment of alpha. In light of the havoc sampling error can wreak

Table 8.9.   Alpha Allocation

Endpoint	Allocation	
Primary	0.040	
Secondary	0.063	
S1		0.035
S2		0.014
S3		0.014
Total	0.100	0.063

as discussed in chapter 1, the need for the *p* value which quantifies sampling error in a decision-making forum is clear. Chapter two provided motivation for us to turn away from the 0.05 standard in favor of intelligently considered alpha apportionment. The PA³S framework provided some guidelines for the prospective allocation of alpha among a collection of prospectively identified primary and secondary endpoints, allowing the investigators to set the terms of the post trial analysis and debate on the findings of each endpoint. Now, we will incorporate the allocation of alpha along asymmetric lines into the development of alpha apportionment, providing needed assurance that the medical ethic of "first do no harm" remains paramount in these complicated experiments with multiple endpoints.

Chapter 6 made ethical arguments for the consideration of thoughtful alpha allocations that are asymmetric. Those arguments are easily folded into PA³S in experiments involving several prospectively defined clinical endpoints. Consider the allocation scheme for a concordantly executed clinical trial with one primary endpoint and four secondary endpoints.

In this circumstance, α_E is set at 0.100, and the maximum acceptable alpha for the primary endpoint is 0.040. Using equation 8.1, α_S is computed to be 0.063. The investigators need to allocate this 0.063 alpha across the three secondary endpoints. Each of the secondary endpoints is of value in this experiment, but the investigators have a stronger sense of concern for S1 and place slightly more alpha there. They divide the remaining alpha between S2 and S3 using equation 8.3. However, how would they now use an asymmetry argument to focus on the possibility of harm?

This may be most directly addressed by dividing the alpha for each endpoint into two components, one measuring the type I error for benefit, the second measuring the harm type I error. If α_p is the allocated alpha for the primary endpoint, then allocate

Table 8.10. PA^{3}S System — Asymmetric Allocation

Endpoint	Allocation		Harm	Benefit
Primary	α_P		$\alpha_P(h)$	$\alpha_P(b)$
Secondary	α_S			
S1		α_{S1}	$\alpha_{S1}(h)$	$\alpha_{S1}(b)$
S2		α_{S2}	$\alpha_{S2}(h)$	$\alpha_{S2}(b)$
S3		α_{S3}	$\alpha_{S2}(h)$	$\alpha_{S2}(b)$
Total	α_E			

Table 8.11. PA^{3}S System — Asymmetric Allocation

Endpoint	Allocation		Harm	Benefit
Primary	0.040		0.025	0.015
Secondary	0.063			
S1		0.035	0.025	0.010
S2		0.014	0.010	0.004
S3		0.014	0.010	0.004
Total	0.100			

$\alpha_p(h)$ for harm and $\alpha_p(b)$ for benefit, such that $\alpha_p(h) + \alpha_p(b) = \alpha_p$. In this example, choosing $\alpha_p(h) = 0.025$, leaves 0.015 for $\alpha_p(b)$. This procedure is repeated for each endpoint in the experiment. This general principle is illustrated in Table 8.10, expanded the alpha allocation table to the right in order to capture the alpha expended for harm and benefit.

The procedure for the investigator to follow is to first choose the total alpha allocation for each endpoint. Then, for each endpoint, divide the total alpha between the benefit and harm tails of the probability distribution. This procedure preserves the total alpha α_E and its apportionment among primary and secondary endpoints, while allowing for the independent ethical placement of alpha for each endpoint.

To elaborate, in the example above we might consider asymmetric alpha allocation as in Table 8.11. The total alpha is conserved at the 0.10 level. The notion of $P_p S_p$, $P_p S_n$, $P_n S_p$, $P_n S_n$ are just as applicable in the asymmetrical alpha apportionment. The trial will be considered positive(benefit) if any of the following occur:

1 the primary endpoint is significant for benefit at the 0.015 level,

2 secondary endpoint S1 is significant for benefit at the 0.010 level,

3 secondary endpoint S2 is significant for benefit at the 0.004 levels.

4 secondary endpoint S3 is significant for benefit at the 0.004 levels.

However, the possibility of harm is more clearly considered and focused in this experiment, and the extension of the vigilant search for harm, reducing the threshold of the strength of scientific evidence used to identify harm, will more likely invoke the of $P^*_p S^*_p$, $P^*_p S_n$, $P_n S^*_p$ descriptors as well. The experiment will be considered positive for harm if:

1 the primary endpoint is significant for harm at the 0.025 level,

2 secondary endpoint S1 is significant for harm at the 0.025 level,

3 secondary endpoint S2 is significant for harm at the 0.010 levels.

4 secondary endpoint S3 is significant for harm at the 0.010 levels.

We should now examine three hypothetical examples of this asymmetric allocation scheme. All three are hypothetical, but are both are taken from real research design concerns.

Asymmetric Example 1 — New Therapy for Hypercholesterolemia

A physician-scientist is developing a compound, which has been described as the next generation of cholesterol lowering therapy. Previous medications had LDL cholesterol as their target of impact the, with only minor changes in HDL cholesterol. The new therapy (Hydyl) targets the HDL cholesterol, promising dramatic increases in HDL cholesterol with no effect on LDL cholesterol levels. Since an objective of lipid modification regimens is reduction in LDL cholesterol and elevation of HDL cholesterol levels, the investigator believes this therapy, when added to current cholesterol reduction regimens, will more favorably adjust patient lipid profiles.

The investigator reviews the community standard of care for

cholesterol level modification. Physicians in general are pleased with the available agents for lipid level adjustments in their patients. Current therapy for cholesterol reduction is well established and, with the introduction of "statin" agents since the 1980s, has provided a range of LDL change that has been well characterized. A patient's response to the current lipid regimen is predictable, with an easily identified, understood, and treatable side effect profile. Thus the standard medications, when used as directed, have provided safe, stable, predictable changes in LDL cholesterol levels. The use of Hydyl should theoretically reduce the occurrence of clinical events related to atherosclerotic disease, providing increased benefit. However, the side effect profile of the new therapy is significant, and patients will need to be observed closely for clinical difficulties, which can include some serious cardiovascular toxic effects, and even death.

To examine the effect of Hydyl, when added to the currently accepted cholesterol reduction regimen, investigators will conduct a prospectively designed, double-blind, placebo-controlled experiment. Each patient will have evidence of atherosclerotic cardiovascular disease, and will be placed (by a random mechanism) on either the standard therapy plus Hydyl, or the standard therapy plus placebo. All patients, regardless of their therapy will be followed for five years to collect data on clinical events. The experiment will have several endpoints. The primary endpoint will be fatal and nonfatal myocardial infarction. Although total mortality is always an important consideration, the investigators believe there will not be enough deaths to be able to draw clear conclusions based on all deaths alone; total mortality will therefore be a secondary endpoint. A third endpoint is the need for revascularization (percutaneous transluminal coronary angioplasty (PTCA) or coronary artery bypass grafts (CABG). Alpha allocation is crucial in this experiment because of the need to consider the differential effect of the therapy across the different endpoints; the investigators recognize that it is possible for the experiment to be negative for the primary endpoint of fatal or nonfatal myocardial infarction but produce positive (benefit) findings for secondary endpoints. In addition, they must give consideration to the possibility of an adverse effect on total mortality, since the therapy is noted to have toxic non-cardiovascular adverse effects.

Alpha allocation begins with the assessment that the current standard of medical care for cholesterol reduction is satisfactory — LDL reduction therapy is well established with a good risk/benefit

Table 8.12.   PA^{3}S System—Asymmetric Allocation—Hydyl Example

Endpoint	Allocation		Harm	Benefit
Primary	0.060		0.050	0.010
Fatal/nonfatal MI				
Secondary	0.069			
Total Mortality		0.065	0.060	0.005
Revascularization		0.004	0.003	0.001
Total	0.125			

profile and a well understood side effect profile. Since the investigators are more interested in the primary endpoint the secondary endpoints, they apportion alpha as 0.060 for the primary endpoint, leaving 0.069 for the secondary endpoints. For the secondary endpoints, they are also concerned with the possibility of harm, and place alpha as in Table 8.12.

The total alpha allocated is 0.125. The investigators require strong evidence for benefit and sensitive protection against harm, so they choose to require a significance test for the primary endpoint at the level of 0.01 level, and 0.05 for harm . Thus, for the primary endpoint, the probability of a type I error must be very small before one can argue for benefit. Accepting a significance test at level greater than 0.01 (say, 0.03) would increase likelihood that the population has produced a sample which has misled the investigators, i.e. the medication is a noxious placebo in the population, but masqueraded as effective in the sample. Such a finding would unleash on the unsuspecting, well-treated population a medication with no efficacy but that produces side effects, an unacceptable state of affairs. However, the investigators are very anxious about a possible harmful effect of therapy, and so require evidence at the 0.05 level to demonstrate that the medication increases the risk of fatal and nonfatal myocardial infarction.

Although much of the interest resides in the primary endpoint, the investigators must consider the findings for secondary endpoints which may be positive as well. They realize that this may be very unlikely in the case of total mortality, since the cumulative total mortality event rate is less than that for the primary endpoint, and the experiment may be underpowered. However, the investigators would still like to identify a prospectively positive finding for the secondary endpoint of total mortality (admitting the goal of $P_p S_p$ or $P_n S_p$). Similarly, they acknowledge that there may be some difficulty interpreting a finding for revascula-

Table 8.13.   PA³S—Asymmetric Allocation Hydyl Trial Results I

Endpoint	Allocation	Harm	Benefit
Primary			0.009
Fatal/nonfatal MI	(0.060)	(0.050)	(0.010)
Secondary	(0.069)		
Total Mortality			0.150
	(0.065)	(0.060)	(0.005)
Revascularization			0.010
	(0.004)	(0.003)	(0.001)
Total	0.125		

rization since it confounds atherosclerotic disease with investigator initiative[13], but is a clinically acceptable endpoint in a trial examining ischemic heart disease. In addition, the cardiovascular community would expect it to be measured. However, the investigator also is concerned about the possibility of harm. The side effect spectrum of this agent suggests that serious toxic cardiovascular adverse events may occur, so there is a focus on total mortality. The investigators state in Table 8.12 that they will accept five times less evidence of harm than he would of benefit (from a alpha allocation perspective) in their concern for mortality. They therefore will not require the same standard of evidence for harm as they would for benefit regarding revascularization.

By tradition, total alpha allocated is large, but so are the dividends. Adequate concern for community safety from both direct harm by the new agent and the occurrence of a type I error for benefit has been afforded. By this allocation, the investigators have affirmed that they wish to consider the experiment positive even if the primary endpoint is negative. The investigators' mandate for alpha allocation has been used to meld a power analysis design and interpretative framework, providing both scientific rigor and community protection.

How would this experiment be interpreted? Consider Table 8.13.

---

[13] The decision to carry out PTCA or CABG is often as much an issue of policy and community practice as it is medical need. Thus, differences in the occurrence rates of these procedures may be due to differences across communities. The random allocation mechanism will distribute community heterogeneity across therapy groups, but it remains a factor which sometimes complicates the generalization of findings of differences of rates of these procedures attributable to the trials tested intervention.

The numbers in parentheses represent the alpha allocations, while the numbers in bold represent the *p* values from the experiment. The findings for the primary endpoint fall in the critical region; the findings for each of the secondary endpoints do not fall in the critical region, so the study is $P_p S_n$. There would be no dispute about these findings, even though the total alpha for the study exceeded 0.05 because the 0.05 level is irrelevant here. What matters is 1) the prospective, ethical alpha allocation and 2) a concordant execution of the experiment. However, other scenarios for this experiment's results are worthy of exploration. For example, the results could have come out as follows:

Table 8.14. PA^3S — Asymmetric Allocation Hydyl Trial Results 2

Endpoint	Allocation		Harm	Benefit
Primary				0.009
Fatal/nonfatal MI	(0.060)		(0.050)	(0.010)
Secondary	(0.069)			
Total Mortality			0.055	
		(0.065)	(0.060)	(0.005)
Revascularization			0.070	
		(0.004)	(0.003)	(0.001)
Total	0.125			

In this scenario, the finding for the primary endpoint was positive for benefit (p value of 0.009 vs. a prior alpha allocation of 0.010). However, the findings for total mortality demonstrate a substantive harmful effect (p value 0.055 vs. a priori alpha of 0.060). The findings for revascularization are not significant (0.070 for harm vs. a priori alpha of 0.003). How should this experiment be interpreted? Using our notation from earlier in this chapter, this experiment would be interpreted as a $P_p S^*_p$ signifying a beneficial therapy effect for the primary endpoint, but a harmful effect of therapy for the secondary endpoint. However, in the final analysis, we look to our credo of "first do no harm" which dictates that this trial be logged as a trial that demonstrated harm, regardless of the beneficial finding for the primary endpoint.

Finally, if the findings were for a positive beneficial effect for the primary endpoint and for total mortality, but a significant, harmful effect for the secondary endpoint of revascularization, the decision to describe this $P_p S_{1p} S^*_{2p}$ result as positive or nega-

Table 8.15. PA^{3}S System — Asymmetric Allocation

Endpoint	Allocation	Harm	Benefit
Exercise Tolerance	0.100	0.075	0.025
Total Mortality	0.006	0.005	0.001
Total	0.106		

tive overall would be difficult. The positive beneficial findings for fatal and nonfatal myocardial infarction and for total mortality would not be adumbrated by the harmful effect of the therapy on revascularization. However, the harmful effect of therapy on the S_2 endpoint would be difficult to ignore. At best, the result would be described as positive but incoherent.[14]

Asymmetric Example 2 — Heart Failure

Consider an investigator who is designing a clinical trial to determine the effect of a compound for congestive heart failure. His primary interest and experience with the drug suggest that it would be most useful as an agent that increases exercise tolerance. However, he is concerned about the possibility of side effects with the drug and wants to monitor total mortality closely. The investigator believes that this compound will not produce any effect on total mortality, but he is not certain. He therefore apportions alpha for this trial as follows.

The total alpha expended for this project is 0.106. The overwhelming majority of this is allocated for the primary endpoint, with 0.025 allocated for benefit, and because of the preeminent concern for harm, expending 0.075 for the possibility of a type I error for harm. The investigator apportions only a small fraction of the available alpha for total mortality, and again allocates a greater alpha for harm. The investigator allocates only a small amount for the important endpoint of total mortality because he

---

[14] Incoherence (3) refers to the finding that the effect of the therapy was inconsistant across the endpoints of the study.

Table 8.16.   PA³S System – Asymmetric Allocation

Endpoint	Allocation	Harm	Benefit
Primary	0.100		
Exercise Tolerance		0.075	0.025
Secondary			
Total Mortality	0.006	0.005	0.001
Total	0.106		

understands that, with the small number of deaths anticipated, he is very unlikely to have any real information about the effect of the therapy on cumulative mortality in the population.

If it is so unlikely that the investigator will capture enough deaths in the sample to be able to make a statement, then why attempt a statement at all? Why apportion alpha where you expect no ability to identify a population effect? One reason is that total mortality is extremely important, perhaps the most important endpoint of a clinical trial. As long as total mortality is a prospective endpoint, the distribution of deaths in the experiment can be a bombshell, and requires some formal prospective attention to avoid experimental discordance. The investigator may very well be surprised by a strong finding for mortality. Consider the following possible results for this investigator.

In this scenario, the finding for the primary endpoint does not fall in the critical region, but the finding for the secondary endpoint is very positive. With a small number of deaths, most all of them occuring in the control group, causing the test statistic for total mortality to fall in the critical region (benefit), the trial is indisputably $P_n S_p$. With a prospective statement concerning identifying total mortality as an endpoint the investigator can draw a clear alpha conserving, noncorrupting conclusion from his experiment based on the secondary endpoint. Without such a statement, the investigator would be subject to severe criticism for drawing a conclusion about total mortality based on post hoc analysis.

This is worth reiterating. The claim of a total mortality benefit in the absence of the prospective statement based on its emergence at the trial's end is clearly data based and experimentally discordant, leading to alpha corruption (see chapter 1). Clearly the investigators would not highlight the unanticipated total mortality finding if it had not been so positive. The alpha allocation

Table 8.17. PA^{3}S—Asymmetric Allocation

Endpoint	Allocation	Harm	Benefit
Total Mortality	0.150	0.100	0.050
Arrhythmic Death	0.100	0.075	0.025
Cardiac Nonarrhythmic Death	0.075	0.050	0.025
Cardiovascular Death	0.075	0.045	0.025
Total	0.345		

scheme of Table (8.16), would allow the investigators to claim P_nS_p with very little a priori alpha penalty.

Asymmetric Example 3—Arrhythmias

For a final example, consider a hypothetical controversial research program. On the heels of CAST[15], use of antiarrhythmic medication development has been understandably and exceedingly cautious. An investigator is interested in designing a clinical experiment that will assess the efficacy of a new antiarrhythmic agent, Dyslyn, in patients who are at serious risk for arrhythmic death. Only patients who have had a recent myocardial infarction with left ventricular deterioration will be recruited for this study. Patients will be randomized to one of two treatment arms: placebo or Dyslyn therapy. The primary endpoint of the experiment is total mortality, with secondary endpoints of arrhythmic death, cardiovascular death, and noncardiovascular death.

The investigator understands that the current treatment of arrhythmias in the postinfarction population is limited by the dearth of available effective medications. If Dyslyn is effective, it will radically change this unacceptably low standard of care. However, the investigator also knows that the preliminary work on Dyslyn has revealed that the medication has serious side effects. Sometimes, it may replace one arrhythmia with another, more deadly one. The investigator chooses to apportion alpha in this setting as follows.

The total alpha for this experiment as designed is 0.345! To

---

[15] Chapter six discusses the CAST trial and the harmful effect antiarrhythmic agents can have.

those who hold fast to the traditional requirement of 0.05 alpha, this apportionment raises deep concerns for the possibility of a type I error in this design. However, here, ethical considerations clearly predominate. The asymmetric approach to alpha allocation is used for each of the four endpoints and, in each case, the concern for harm garners most of the alpha allocated. Of the 0.150 alpha allocated for the total mortality endpoint, 0.100 is allocated for harm and 0.050 allocated for benefit, consistent with the overriding concern about the possibility of harm. However, the investigators also want to insure that they not miss the promise of a beneficial effect. This perspective is justified by the poor standard of community care for arrhythmic care and is exemplified in the investigator's allocation of as much as 0.050 for the total mortality benefit and 0.025 for each of arrhythmic death, cardiac non-arrhythmic death, and cardiovascular death. Since the small number of arrhythmic deaths, and deaths in the other cause specific mortality categories will blunt his ability to identify effects in this sample which are due to more than just sampling error, the investigator wishes to prospectively formulate a plan which would allow him to identify a beneficial effect of therapy for either arrhythmic death, cardiac non-arrhythmic death, or cardiovascular death, even though such a finding is unlikely with the lower event rates.

Still, the total alpha outlay, 0.345, is large. This means that globally there is a one chance in three that efficacy in the sample does not reflect efficacy in the population through chance alone. Is this large alpha outlay acceptable? The investigator can make a solid case for this generous alpha allocation, beginning with a description of the environment in which the experiment will be conducted. Clinicians are hard pressed to identify useful therapy for these patients who are seriously ill. The investigator therefore does not which to miss a beneficial effect, and is willing to run an increased risk of deciding in favor of therapy even if in fact no effect is seen in the population. He decides the increased risk of type I error on the side of benefit is appropriate.

However, the findings of the possibility of harm in previous research require the investigator to also concentrate on the very real likelihood that harm will befall these patients. Previous work to date suggests that patients may be at increased risk of death due to the use of agents like Dyslyn. The investigator wishes to provide adequate assurance that, if this is the case, the experiment would be sensitive enough to identify it. The investigator is fighting a two-front war, confronting on the one hand the real specter of harm while simultaneously evaluating the possibility of establishing a dramatic improvement in the standard of care for cardiac arrhythmias. The alpha allocation here is justifiable for this sensitive experiment.

He provides this sensitivity by (1) using asymmetric bounds for the type I error and (2) having adequate type I error for each endpoint. The physician-scientists will be examining, treating, and following these patients in this trial will have the assurance that appropriate attention to the possibly of harm has been embedded in the experiment. This attention is translated into a sensitive and intelligent allocation of type I alpha, reflecting the heightened concern for harm.

This prospective allocation scheme admits a number of interesting and provocative conclusions about the trial. Of course, the investigator desires to see P_pS_p or P_pS_n positivity. However, the selection of secondary endpoints, with prospective alpha allocated for each of them, suggests the likelihood of P_nS_p positivity. The study could be considered positive if the findings for total mortality were negative, but there was benefit for any of the three cause-specific mortality endpoints. arrhythmic death, cardiac non-arrhythmic death, and cardiovascular death. However, the investigator must admit that there is a possibility of a $P_nS^*_p$ finding, e.g., the trial is negative for total mortality but demonstrates a harmful effect on cardiac nonarrhythmic death. The "first do no harm" principle requires that this trial be documented as demonstrating this harmful effect of the therapy. Is it possible the trial could be positive (benefit) for total mortality, and, at the same time be positive (harm) for cardiac non-arrhythmic death? Certainly, a $P_pS^*_p$ finding is possible. However, I believe such an event would be unlikely, since the patients recruited would be those who are most at risk for arrhythmic death and there would be relatively few non-cardiac arrhythmic deaths. Still, the primary ethic of medicine would require this trial prominently highlight this unfortunate finding.

Extending from the definition of a positive trial as one that is positive for the primary endpoint to include those that which are negative for the primary endpoint but positive for secondary endpoints can only be seen as a relaxation of the criteria for positive trials. This relaxation comes at the acceptable price of tightening secondary endpoint interpretation standards. In the author's experience, secondary endpoint decision rules are handled cursorily (if at all) in the design phase of a randomized controlled clinical trial. Only at the end of the experiment is there a scramble to "put the right spin" on their interpretation. It is best to reject this approach to secondary endpoint management. Secondary endpoints should be considered positive only if an alpha allocation scheme (PA³S or another) is applied to them and rigorously followed in their interpretation. The customary standard for secondary endpoints is very weak; I suggest that we raise it, balancing this increase in standard by opening the door for a disciplined interpretation scheme admitting $P_n S_p$ trials as positive.

Certainly, the use of a prospective allocation scheme has not solved all of the problems in designing this ethically delicate experiment. The important consideration here is that under PA³S, there is the opportunity to review the results of the experiment without the alpha corruption concerns that typically adumbrate the trial conclusions in the absence of prospective alpha allocation for secondary endpoints. PA³S has provided a framework in which each of these concerns can be addressed. It has provided the construct for the clear delineation of the possibility of harm in each endpoint. It has also sparked a debate and hopefully a consensus in the cardiology community for the types of concerns for the various endpoints of the study. Finally, it has appropriately set the terms of the posttrial debate. It has precisely defined the rules for judging the trial to be a success, minimizing the likelihood of experimental discordance for endpoint determination and critical region to corrupt the type I and type II errors.

Type I error Dependency

The presence of dependent hypothesis tests induced by endpoint-set correlation (dependency) can result in generous alpha allocation[15]. This consideration is dependency is admissible if 1) there is biologic plausibility for the nature of the dependency and 2) the investigators make a reasonable prospective statement on the magnitude of the dependency. In such circumstances, the adjustment presented here is an over-adjustment, leading to alpha levels lower than required, and the incorporation of a dependency argument can lead to an important savings in alpha allocation. However, the inclusion of such a dependency term can lead to a substantial reduction in alpha expense. This presumes the nature of

Table 8.18. Alpha error dependency in clinical trial design

		Primary Endpoint		
		Type I Error	No Type I Error	Total
Secondary	Type I Error	0.02	0.005	0.025
Endpoint	No Type I Error	0.005	0.97	0.975
	Total	0.025	0.975	1.000

the dependency is clear, quantifiable and defensible. However, perhaps this is an overstatement of the problem. A clinical trial[16] that made prospective arguments for dependency among the collection of primary and secondary events was successfully presented and defended a Federal Food and Drug Administration public hearing in February 1997. This led to the computation of an alpha based on both primary and secondary endpoints that kept the overall alpha spent below an acceptable upper bound.

As a further elaboration on the impact of a dependency argument in alpha allocation, consider the implications of correlation between the likelihood of a Type I error for two co-primary endpoints (Table 8.18).

In this case, the total alpha expended is $1 - 0.97 = 0.03$. By assuming the test on the primary endpoint is independent of the test on the secondary endpoint, the Type I error expended is $1 - (0.025)(0.025) = 0.0494$. When compared to the expenditure of 0.03 using the dependency argument, the incorporation of dependency led to a $100^*(0.0494 - 0.030)/0.0494 = 39.2$ percent savings.

Alpha Eggs in the Endpoint Basket

Choosing among correlated endpoints and placing them in a primary or secondary position, may seem counterproductive. Unfortunately, the current state of affairs represents an extreme position, because artificial categorization of correlated endpoints is the current norm. Commonly, one endpoint is chosen as the primary endpoint from among a collection of correlated endpoints and all

---

[16] This clinical trial examined the impact of integrilin in the immediate postpercutaneous transluminal coronary angioplasty (PTCA) setting.

alpha is expended on it; the remaining correlated endpoints are essentially ignored. This reflects the ultimate in artificial categorization, and as an extreme example of a counterproductive decision process. Yet it is PA³S which allows us to move away from this unfortunate extreme. Under PAAS, alpha can be applied prospectively and differentially to each of the correlated endpoints, allowing each endpoint to make a contribute to the decision process and avoiding the requirement of placing all alpha "eggs" in one primary endpoint "basket."

Conclusions

The propositions offered in this chapter are based on the preeminent need to protect the scientific and patient communities from dangerous type I errors, errors that could result, for example from the new availability to patients of ineffective compounds with nontrivial side effects—compounds promulgated as "safe and effective," but which are actually noxious placebos. However, the change in alpha policy advocated here is sensitive to the needs of statisticians, physician-scientists, regulatory agencies, industry, and the patient community.

Strategies for *p* value interpretation have been offered in the past.[17] Here I advocate a change in alpha policy which encourages prospective alpha allocations for many clinical experiments. This change in policy has two components. The first is an improvement in the scientific community standard for prospective statements about alpha, requiring clear alpha allocations for primary and secondary endpoints. The second is a differentiation between the experimental alpha, α_E and the alpha allocated for the primary endpoint, α_P. A consequence of the proposed approach is, that, since alpha will be expended on secondary endpoints, less alpha can be expended on the primary endpoint in order to constrain the alpha of the experiment at an acceptable upper bound. Thus, adequately powered experiments with secondary endpoints will pay a price for these endpoints' interpretation (an increased sample size for the $\alpha_P < 0.05$). Many workers will understandably react negatively to this consequence. Yet, if

---

[17] See Chapter 6.

the secondary endpoint is to have an objective interpretation, this interpretation must occur in the context of the alpha expended.

In response to these concerns, based on arguments proposed in chapter 2, I also suggest that α_E be set to a value greater than 0.05, allowing investigators liberal alpha to distribute among secondary endpoints. Secondary endpoints add considerable strength to the findings of an experiment. If many endpoints are positive in the same direction, the trial is consistent, its several endpoints speaking with one voice. Investigators need not be penalized for including devices, such as secondary endpoints that add to trial efficiency and coherency. Allowing a considerable difference between α_E and α_P permits ample opportunity for positive findings for secondary endpoints. The payoff for investigators is the new admissibility of $P_n S_p$ positivity.

In addition, I recognize is the assessment of a clinical trial which is negative for the primary endpoint but has positive findings either for secondary endpoints or in post hoc analyses can be very frustrating. Perhaps the interpretation of these experiments should be contentious. Part of the difficulty lies in the terminology of clinical trial interpretation. Words such as positive and negative are useful but coarse. This chapter introduced the notion of a prospective assymetric alpha allocation scheme (PA^{3}S), introducing trial result descriptions in terms of trial endpoints. The combination of a prospective allocation argument, new terminology, and the incorporation of asymmetric alpha allocation provides the setting in which an experiment that does not reject the null hypothesis for the primary endpoint but does reject the null hypothesis for secondary endpoints may be considered positive. In addition, an argument is made for differentiating between the Type I error of the experiment (α_E) and the total type I error for the primary endpoint(s), α_P, serves the useful purpose of conserving sample size, incorporating thoughtful consideration of ethics, and preserving consistency with past standards of strength of evidence for the primary endpoint of clinical trials.

Is the conservative approach to type I error always necessary? Certainly not. In pilot studies, and in endeavors that are exploratory, stringent alpha management is not required, and ultraconservatism may be counterproductive. However, when a new type of care is developed for a patient population, exposing these patients to compounds and interventions with significant side effects, alpha management is essential. Far from being a pernicious abstraction, tight alpha conservatism is required to avoid population exposure to noxious placebos.

The contribution of PA³S is that it represents one step forward from the current, amorphous "don't ask, don't tell" policy for multiple endpoint a priori alpha allocations. Moreover, PA³S represents a step forward that does not require clinical trialists to accept the ultralow alpha levels that often result from the application of Bonferoni's approximation. However, attempting to manipulate the prospective choice of an alpha level solely to "win" (i.e., with the sole motivation to get the test statistic for the primary endpoint into the critical region), denigrates the entire process, regardless of which system for alpha allocation is used. Any prospectively chosen alpha levels should be set based on the notion of community protection. Alpha designations made for example, to prevent the exposure of the community to noxious placebo would add a much-needed clinical dimension to what is a commonly perceived as a sterile, artificial, mathematical metric. Like the choice of an endpoint, the choice of prospective alpha levels should also be based on prospective clinical reasoning and concern for community protection.

Of course there are scholarly alternatives to the PA³S system — this chapter refers to several of them. Each alternative is valid, but each has the weakness of its strength. Because they are complex, they are fairly incomprehensible to non-statisticians. We must keep sight of the fact that, in contemporary society, weighing the evidence from research efforts is no longer the isolated purview of technical specialists. Today, data are reviewed by regulators, legislators, practicing physicians, and, in these litigious times, judges and juries as well. Many of these decision makers can understand the underlying principle of sample based research and the role of *p* values in assessing the impact of sampling error on a research conclusion.

This begs the question, how are these nonquantitative experts to draw conclusions in this complicated research environment? It is unfortunate that the legislators, judges, regulators and physicians who must draw conclusions from sample based research cannot wait for the future blossoms of statistical research efforts while they hold tightly in their hands the thorns of today's research controversies. We as statisticians must provide tools that are useful, informative, intuitive, and consistent with the fundamental tenet of sample based research: first — say what you plan to do, then do what you said. Systems like PA³S meet these criteria.

References

1. Snedecor, G.W., and Cochran, W.G., (1980) *Statistical Methods*, 7th Edition Iowa State University Press.
2. Moyé, L.A., (1998) "P value Interpretation and Alpha Allocation in Clinical Trials," *Annals of Epidemiology* 8:351–357.
3. Pfeffer, M.A., Braunwald, E., Moyé, L.A., Basta, L., Brown, E.J., Cuddy, T.E., Davis, B.R., Geltman, E.M., Goldman, S., Flaker, G.C., Klein, M., Lamas, G.A., Packer, M., Rouleau, J., Rouleau, J.L., Rutherford, J., Wertheimer, J.H., and Hawkins, C.M. for the SAVE Investigators (1992) "Effect of Captopril on mortality and morbidity in patients with left ventricular dysfunction after myocardial infarction—results of the Survival and Ventricular Enlargement Trial," *New England Journal of Medicine* 327:669–677.
4. Sacks, F.M., Pfeffer, M.A., Moyé, L.A., Louleau, J.L., Rutherford, J.D., Cole, T.G., Brown, L., Warnica, J.W., Arnold, J.M.O., Wun, C.C., Davis, B.R., and Braunwald, E., (1996) for the Cholestrol and recurrent Events Trial Investigators. 1996. "The effect of pravastatin on coronary events after myocardial infarction in patients with average cholesterol levels," *New England Journal of Medicine* 335:1001–1009.
5. The Sytolic Hypertension in the Elderly Program (SHEP) Co-operative Research Group. (1991) "Prevention of Stroke by Antihypertensive Drug Therapy in Older Persons with Isolated Systolic Hypertension: Final Results of the Systolic Hypertension in the Elderly Program (SHEP)," *Journal of the American Medical Association* 265:3255–3264.
6. Mahmarian, J.J., Moyé, L.A., Chinoy, D.A., Sequeira, R.F., Habib, G.B., Henry, W.J., Jain, A., Chaitman, B.R., Weng, C.S.W., Morales-Ballejo, H., and Pratt, C.M., (1998) "Transdermal nitroglycerin patch therapy improves left ventricular function and prevents remodeling after acute myocardial infarction: results of a multicentre prospective randomized double-blind placebo controlled trial," *Circulation* 97:2017–2024.
7. The LRC Investigators. (1984) "The Lipid Research Clinics Coronary Primary Prevention trial results," *Journal of the American Medical Association* 251:351–374.
8. Cardiac Arrhythmia Suppression Trial (CAST) Investigators. "Preliminary report: effect of encainide and flecanide on mortality in a randomized trial of arrhythmia suppression after myocardial infarction," *New England Journal of Medicine* 321:227–233.
9. Linet, M.S., Hatch, E.E., Kleinerman, R.A., Robison, L.L., Kaune, W.T., Freidman, D.R., Severson, R.K., Haines, C.M., Hartsock, C.T., Niwa, S., Wacholder, S., and Tarone, R.E., (1997) "Residential Exposure to Magnetic Fields and acute lymphoblastic leukemia in children," *New England Journal of Medicine* 337:1–7.

10. Hayes, D.L., Wang, P.J., Reynolds, D.W., Estes, M., Griffith, J.L., Steffens, R.A., Carlo, G.L., Findlay, G.K., and Johnson, C.M., (1997) "Interference with cardiac pacemakers by cellular telephones," *New England Journal of Medicine* 336:1473–1479.

11. Westfall, P.H., and Young, S., "P value adjustments for multiple tests in multivariate binomial models," *Journal of the American Statistical Association* 84:780–786.

12. Lan, K.K.G., and Demets, D.L., (1983) "Discrete sequential boundaries for clinical trials," *Biometrika*, 70:659–663.

13. Lan, K.K.G., Simon, R., and Halperin, M. (1982) "Stochastically curtailed tests in long-term clinical trials," *Communications in Statistics* C1:207–209.

14. Davis, B.R., and Hardy, R.J., (1990) "Upper bounds for type I and type II error rates in conditional power calculations," *Communications in Statistics* 19:3571–3584.

15. Lan, K.K.G., and Wittes, J., (1988) "The b-value: a tool for monitoring data". *Biometrics*, 44:579–585.

16. Wesfall, P.H., Krishnen, A., and Young S., (1998) "Using prior information to allocate significance levels for multiple endpoints," *Statistics in Medicine* 17:2107–2119.

9

CHAPTER

Neurons vs. Silicon: Regression Analysis and *P* values

The New Meaning of Regression

Regression analysis is everywhere in medical statistical inference, and so are its *p* values. Its omnipresence comes as no real surprise. At their core, regression analysis and health care research are about relationship examination (e.g., does a new therapy for hypertension improve clinical outcomes?) In medicine we want to understand what either causes or cures diseases and we learn about these causes through exploring relationships. Regression analysis is the statistical tool that allows us a quantitative view of these relationships. This chapter's purpose is not to teach regression analysis[1] but, after a brief review, to develop a disciplined approach to *p* value incorporation and interpretation in its use.

Much of the statistical analysis in health care today falls under the rubric of regression analysis. Its explosive growth has been fueled by the computational devices that have evolved over the last forty years. Increasingly affordable computing stations and software, once only within the reach of the statistical specialist, are now being wielded by nonstatisticians. In addition, regression analysis procedures themselves have expanded so that they have subsumed other modes of analysis traditionally viewed as related

---

[1] I assume that the reader has had a brief exposure to regression analysis in an introductory course in statistics.

to but separate from regression analysis. Initially, regression analysis was designed to look at the relationship between two variables, a dependent variable whose value the investigator was interested in predicting and a single independent variable used to "explain" the dependent variable. In classical regression analysis, both of these variable were continuous variables.[2] However, the development of computing techniques and theory have led to a dramatic expansion from this paradigm. Models that have more than one independent variable are commonly examined (in what is still known as multiple regression analysis). Also, regression analysis now includes the examination of relationships between a continuous dependent variable and polychotamous independent variables (formally known as the analysis of variance), as well as also between a continuous dependent variable and a mixture of polychotamous and continuous independent variables (also known as the analysis of covariance). Repeated measure analysis allows each subject to have multiple measurements obtained over the course of time to be analyzed. Complicated models mixing within subjects and between subject effects are also now contained within the domain of regression analysis. In addition, the dependent variable could be dichotomous (logistic regression analysis), or represent information that reflects survival (Cox regression analysis). In fact, the simple two sample *t* test introduced in an introductory course in statistics and most commonly not taught as a regression problem can in fact be completed derived and understood as a result from regression analysis.

Thus, through its expansion, regression analysis is now a common analysis in health care, and is commonly carried out by non-statisticians. It is a procedure that produces tremendous reams (or screens) of results. Each independent variable in each model, produces a *p* value. *P* values are produced in main effect models, for interaction terms, and for covariates. *P* values can be used for unadjusted effects, and adjusted effects. The giant software engines of the 21st century belch forth these *p* values by the tens and by the hundreds. The purpose of this chapter is to express the philosophy of model building and *p* value interpretation in regression analysis problems in health care. Unless great care is taken in this inter-

---

[2] A continuous variable e.g., age permits integer and fraction values. A dichotomous variable has only two levels (e.g., male and female). A polychotamous variable has multiple levels but no particular value is placed on the order (e.g.,1-white, 2-African-American, 3-hispanic, 4-oriental).

pretation, misleading results can be obtained. We will appreciate that the greater the computer "silicon's" tendency to spew out p values, the stronger our "neurons" (i.e., our intellectual discipline) must be.

Underlying Assumptions in Simple Regression Analysis

The hallmark of regression analysis is relationship exploration. In health care, this relationship dissection can be exploited to predict the value of the dependent, (unknown) variable from the value of the independent (known) variable. The most common motivation for examining relationships between variables in health care is the construction of a causality argument. As we recall, the tenets of causality have many non statistical components, i.e., criteria other than a single analysis relating the putative risk factor to the disease. The correct use of regression analysis in a well-designed experiment will provide solid support to the arguments that address these tenets, helping to construct a solid causality argument. However, in order to be convincing, this regression building block must be precisely engineered.

This is one of the motivations for a clear understanding of the assumptions underlying regression analysis. We begin with a straightforward model in regression analysis, the simple straight line model. Assume we have collected n pairs of observations (x_i, y_i), i = 1 to n. Our goal is to demonstrate that changes in the value of x are associated with changes in the value of y. We will assume that x and y are linearly related. From this we write the simple linear regression model

$$E[y_i] = \beta_0 + \beta_1 x_i$$

This is the statement that the dependent variable y is a linear function of x's. The larger the value of the coefficient β_1, the stronger the linear relationship between x and y. In regression analysis, we assume that the beta coefficients are parameters whose true values we will never know since that would require including everyone in the population in our experiment. We will estimate parameters β_0 and β_1 with parameter estimates b_0 and b_1 respectively. The estimates we will use are called least square estimates. These estimates are unbiased, and have the smallest variance of any unbiased estimators that are linear functions of the dependent variable. In order to predict the expected value of y in this model, we will make some common assumptions. They are that

1) The model is correct.

It serves no purpose to exert time and energy into collecting data and performing an analysis if the underlying relationship between x and y is wrong. It pays to explore the literature and gain experience with the variables in the system before making an underlying assumption about the model. In this example, if the relationship between x and y is not a straight-line relationship, our modeling results are DOA (dead on arrival).

2) The error terms are independent, have common variance, and are normally distributed.

Despite the rigor of the experimental design, and despite the large size of the dataset, it is extremely unlikely that each observation's dependent variable will be predicted by that observation's independent variable. Thus, for our dataset the equation of interest is

$$y_i = b_0 + b_1 x_i + e_i,$$

where e_i is the error term. Just as in a sample of data, the sample mean will not be exactly equal to the population mean, in regression analysis, the sample parameter estimates b_0 and b_1 will not exactly equal the parameters β_0 and β_1. We assume that the error terms e_I are independent, with common variance σ^2. This is the most common assumption in regression analysis, although in some advanced models, this assumption can be relaxed, opening up a wider range of useful experimental designs for which this can be implemented. For the sake of all our hypothesis testing, we will assume the e_I's follow a normal distribution. However, the normality assumption is not required for parameter estimation.

Model Estimation

Let's begin with the model for simple linear regression

$$E[y_i] = \beta_0 + \beta_1 x_i.$$

Since the β's are parameters that can only be known by an analysis of every subject in the population, we attempt to estimate the parameters by drawing a sample (x_i, y_i), $i = \{1, \ldots, n\}$. Our job is to then estimate the β_0 and β_1 by b_0 and b_1 from the n equations $y_i = b_0 + b_1 x_i + e_i$, $i = \{1, \ldots, n\}$ where the e_I are the error terms assumed to follow a standard normal distribution with mean zero and variance σ^2. The errors are also assume to be uncorrelated. Even for a small dataset, having to compute the regression coefficients on a hand calculator is at best inconvenient. Fortunately, statistical software has evolved which is easy to use, it spares us the computational burden, and is almost always accurate in performing the calculation for us.

Simple Examples and Explanations

Consider the following observational study as an example in regression analysis. Two thousands patients are randomly chosen from a population of patients who recently (within the last two weeks) sustained a heart attack. The investigator is interested in looking at predictors of left ventricular dysfunction. Therefore, at baseline, the investigator collects a substantial amount of information on these patients, including demographic information, measures of morbidity prevalence, and measures of heart function. The investigator begins with a small model that predicts left ventricular ejection fraction (*LVEF*) from age i.e., he is "regressing" LVEF on age. The model is

$$E[LVEF_i] = \beta_0 + \beta_1 \, age_i.$$

where E[*LVEF*] means the average value of LVEF. In this model the investigator is assuming that the average LVEF is a straight line function of age. He obtains the following results from his favorite software program (Table 9.1.)

The parameter estimate ($\pm$ its standard error or standard deviation) for b_0 is 33.59 ± 0.81 and for b_1 is -0.043 ± 0.013.

Table 9.1. Univariate Analysis: Regression of LVEF on Age

Variable	Parameter Estimate	Standard Error	T statistic	P Value
INTERCEPT (b_0)	33.593044	0.80979366	41.483	0.0001
AGE (b_1)	−0.043169	0.01342332	−3.216	0.0013

Already, we have p values. The p value for each parameter is a test of the null hypothesis that the parameter is equal to zero. We see that for each of these, the test statistic is large and the p values are small.

Of course it would be a mistake to conclude that this analysis proves that age produces a smaller ejection fraction. Any comment that states or implies causality must be buttressed by arguments addressing the causality tenets[3], arguments that we have not posited here. Similarly, this analysis does not imply that as patients age, they are more likely to have a smaller ejection fraction. We must keep in mind the subtle but important distinction that to make such a longitudinal conclusion would require that we would have to follow a cohort of patients over time, serially measuring their ages and their ejection fractions. That is not the case here; no patient has their ejection fraction measured twice. Instead, a sample of patients was taken and examined in a "snapshot." For each patient, one and only one age was obtained and, for each patient, one and only one ejection fraction was measured. Thus, for this group, we can say only that there is a relationship between a patient's age and their ejection fraction, in that older patients appear to have lower ejection fractions than younger patients. Note the passive tone of this comment. We cannot say that age generates lower ejection fractions or that aging produces smaller LVEF's. We can only say that patients who were older were found to have smaller ejection fractions on average than patients who were younger. This careful distinction in the characterization of this relationship is a trait of the disciplined researcher who uses regression analysis.

What does the p value of 0.0013 mean? Using our community protection oriented definition, it means that it is very unlikely that a postinfarction population in which there is no relationship between ejection fraction and patient age would produce a sample in which this relationship is identified. However, the small p value contributes very little to a causality argument here. Since, of course, age cannot be assigned randomly to an individual, we cannot be sure that it is really age to which the ejection fraction is related. Other possible explanations for this LVEF–age relationship is that older patients may have had more than one heart attack; perhaps it is the number of heart attacks that is really re-

---

[3] The Bradford Hill causality tenets are discussed in chapter 3.

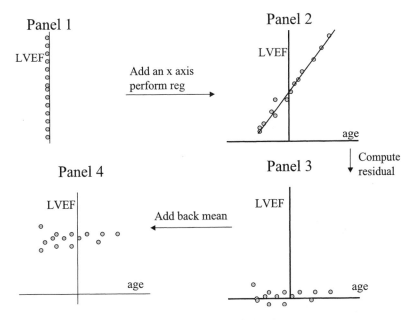

Figure 9.1. Step-by-step view of regression

lated to ejection fraction. Thus, we can only say that it appears that age and LVEF are related.[4] This is by necessity a very weak message.

Variance Partitioning

Before we move onto the examination of another variable in this cross sectional analysis, it would be useful to explain the mathematics underlying the construction of the LVEF-age relationship. Regression analysis is a form of variance examination. We can follow this variance in LVEF as we go through the process of modeling LVEF as a function of age. If we start the analysis, measuring only the ejection fraction and no other explanatory variable, we see the anticipated scatter in the LVEF's across patients (Figure 9.1 Panel 1).

This is anticipated—we say that the total variability in ejection fraction is unexplained. We attribute it all to sampling error and

---

[4] The difficulty of assigning a reason for an effect when the supposed reason is not assigned randomly is discussed in chapter 3.

write the total variability of the system as

$$Total\ Variability = \sum_{i=1}^{n}(y_i - \bar{y})^2$$

However, it is possible that another variable would "explain" some of the variability or the spread of the ejection fractions across patients. We intelligently choose to measure age and we see that the total variability that we recognized in panel one can be divided into two components. The first is the component that we say is due to the regression, i.e., the variation in ejection fraction due to variation in the age of the patients. However, there is still variation which is unexplained. This unexplained, or residual variation is seen graphically as the vertical distance from each point to the straight line representing the relationship between the ejection fraction and age (Panel 2). This is depicted algebraically as

$$Total\ Variability = \sum_{i=1}^{n}(y_i - \bar{y})^2 = \sum_{i=1}^{n}(y_i - \hat{y}_i + \hat{y}_i - \bar{y})^2$$
$$= \sum_{i=1}^{n}((y_i - \hat{y}_i) + (\hat{y}_i - \bar{y}))^2$$

by going through the multiplication of this last expression we find

$$\sum_{i=1}^{n}((y_i - \hat{y}_i) + (\hat{y}_i - \bar{y}))^2 = \sum_{i=1}^{n}(y_i - \hat{y}_i)^2 + \sum_{i=1}^{n}(\hat{y}_i - \bar{y})^2$$
$$+ 2\sum_{i=1}^{n}((y_i - \hat{y}_i)(\hat{y}_i - \bar{y}))^2$$

That last complicated term on the right turns out to be zero. Thus, we have

$$\sum_{i=1}^{n}(y_i - \bar{y})^2 = \sum_{i=1}^{n}(y_i - \hat{y}_i)^2 + \sum_{i=i}^{n}(\hat{y}_i - \bar{y})^2$$

We see algebraically what was produced graphically in figure 9.1. The total variability of the system is broken into two components. The first is the variation in LVEF (y) which is explained by age (x). This variability is termed the sum of squares regression (SSR) and is that component of the total variability that is explained by the regression line. The second is the remaining or residual unexplained variability. It is often called the "sum of squares error"

(SSE) reflecting the degree to which the fitted values deviate from the actual values. In regression analysis, using the least squares approach, we choose the estimates b_0, and b_1 for β_0 and β_1 to minimize the sum of squares error. Since the sum of squares total (SST) is a constant, the least squares approach minimizes SSE and maximizes SSR. An interesting quantity to keep track of in model building is $R^2 = SSR/SST$. This may be thought of as the percent of the total variability explained by the regression model. The range of this measure is from 0 to 1. Models that fit the data well are characterized by small SSE, large SSR, and large R^2. Models that fit the data poorly have large SSEs, small SSRs, and low R^2. If you hope to draw inferential conclusions from models, you are more persuasive if you draw these conclusions from models with large R^2.

Panel 3 is an examination of the residue of the regression analysis. Here we subtract from the LVEF of each patient the LVEF predicted by that patient's age. If the best relationship between LVEF and age is a straightline, panel 3 depicts what the residuals look like. They have a mean value of zero, and variance smaller than the total variance from panel 1. Note that we are focusing on variance of LVEF (vertical variance) and not the variance of the ages (horizontal variance). We would expect this, since much of the variability in LVEF was due to age. Adding back the mean LVEF gives us the location and scatter of the LVEF with the age component removed as depicted in Panel 4.

Enter Dichotomous Independent Variables

The investigator now wishes to examine the relationship between LVEF and the presence of multiple myocardial infarctions (MIs, or heart attacks). His suspicion is that patients with multiple heart attacks will have a smaller ejection fractions. However, unlike the independent variable age, which was continuous, the multiple MI variable takes on only two values, zero and one.[5] The flexibility of

---

[5] In fact the examination of the relationship between left ventricular ejection fraction and multiple myocardial infarctions is really an unpaired t-test. The univariate regression to be executed here will give the exact same result as the t-test would.

Table 9.2. Univariate Analysis: Regression of LVEF on Multiple
Myocardial Infarction

Variable	Parameter Estimate	Standard Error	T statistic	P Value
INTERCEPT (b_0)	31.845726	0.17482486	182.158	0.0001
Multiple MI's (b_1)	−2.300272	0.29342045	−7.840	0.0001

regression analysis allows us to incorporate these classes of independent variables as well. In doing so, we can apply everything
we have learned about regression analysis parameter estimates.
However, we will need to very careful about how we interpret the
parameter in this model.

For the model we are examining, y_i is the ejection fraction of
the ith patient, and x_i reflect the presence of multiple myocardial
infarctions, $x_i = 0$ if there are no multiple MI's (i.e., the heat attack
which made the patient eligible for the trial was the patient's first
heart attack, and $x_i = 1$ if the patient has had multiple heart
attacks. Now write the model

$$E[y_i] = \beta_0 + \beta_1 x_i$$

Before we go any further, let's consider the implications of this
model. We have modeled the LVEF as a function of multiple myocardial infarctions. For patients with only one MI, $x_i = 0$, and,
regardless of the value of β_1, the term which contains x_i will be
zero. Thus, for patients with only one MI

$$E[y_i] = \beta_0.$$

For patients with multiple myocardial infarctions, $x_i = 1$, and
their expected left ventricular ejection fraction is

$$E[y_i] = \beta_0 + \beta_1.$$

Thus, β_1 is the difference in the expected LVEF between patients
with only one heart attack and patients with multiple heart attacks. A hypothesis test carried out on β_1 by examining the
parameter estimate b_1 is a test on the impact of multiple MIs on
LVEF in a population of patients with at least one heart attack.
The results of this analysis appear in Table 9.2.

This data reveals that patients with multiple myocardial infarctions in general have an ejection fraction that is 2.30 ± 0.29
(parameter estimate ± its standard error) units less than patients

with only one heart attack. However, we cannot conclude that multiple MI's are the cause of lower ejection fractions. One important reason for this is that the value of the multiple heart attack variable is not assigned randomly. It is associated with many clinical factors, such as longstanding atherosclerotic disease, hypertension, or genetic influences. However, the lack of random assignment of the multiple MI variable to patients (of course this is impossible), precludes the clear attribution of ejection fraction differences to the presence of multiple heart attacks. We can say only that the presence of a multiple MIs is associated with lower ejection fraction, i.e., patients with multiple heart attacks have on average lower ejection fractions than patients with only one heart attack.

Multiple Regression and the Meaning of "Adjustment"

Each of these univariate models had provided an important piece of information involving the influences on left ventricular ejection fraction. However, the two independent variables, age and multiple myocardial infarctions are related. Patients who are older are more likely to have had multiple myocardial infarctions than younger patients. How can the investigator decide which of the two is the driving variable in influencing LVEF?

Regression models with more than one independent variable are commonly considered models which provide adjusted effects for the independent variables. However, words like "adjustment" have very broad uses in science, so we must be precise when we use them in regression analysis. Consider the previous model focusing on the change in LVEF. We know that patients with different values for the multiple heart attack variable will on average have different ages (patients with multiple MI's tend to be older than patients with only one MI) and that age is itself related to LVEF. How can we get at the actual relationship between age and LVEF? One way to do this would be to "hold multiple MI age "constant." That would be tantamount to choosing patients in the sample who have the same value for the multiple myocardial infarction variable but different ages. While this may be reasonable in some cases, it is in general an impractical solution, especially

Table 9.3.   Univariate Analysis: Regression of LVEF on Multiple Myocardial Infarction

Variable	Parameter Estimate	Standard Error	T statistic	P Value
Intercept (b_0)	33.723202	0.80003558	42.152	0.0001
Age (b_1)	−0.032079	0.01333992	−2.405	0.0163
Multiple MI's (b_2)	−2.222026	0.29490668	−7.535	0.0001

when both independent variables are continuous, or there are more than two independent variables.

Consider instead the following results the investigator has obtained by regressing LVEF on both age and the multiple MI variable simultaneously. The model is

$$E\,[\text{LVEF}] = \beta_0 + \beta_1(\text{age}) + \beta_2(\text{multiple MI variable}).$$

From the data in Table 3 which reflects the results of this model. Here each variable appears to have a notable relationship with left ventricular ejection fraction. However, if we compare coefficients across the Tables 9.1, 9.2, and 9.3, we find that the relationships seem to be different in size. The coefficient estimate b_1 for the univariate relationship between LVEF and age (−0.043 from Table 9.1) is different from the estimate in the multiple variable regression (−0.032 Table 9.3) Similarly, we see that −2.300 as the regression estimate b_1 from the univariate model from Table 9.2, but −2.222 is the estimate from for the multiple regression model Table 9.3. What do the new coefficient estimates mean, and which should be reported?

In order to understand the implications of the multiple regression parameter estimates from Table 9.3, we need to examine how these coefficient estimates were obtained. Consider the relationship between LVEF and age. The underlying theory collapses these computations into three stages to compute the estimate from Table 9.3.

1 regress LVEF on multiple MI and compute the residual of LVEF,

2 regress age on multiple MI and compute the residual of age,

3 regress the LVEF residual on the age residual.

These computations are carried out automatically by most regression software. If we were to go through each of these three

Table 9.4. Explicit Regression following three step process LVEF residual on Age residual

Variable	Parameter Estimate	Standard Error	T statistic	P Value
AGE (b_1)	−0.03209	0.01333693	−2.405	0.0162

individual steps ourselves, we would find the result. (Table 4) which matches perfectly with the results from Table 9.3, and now tells us how to interpret the results of the multiple regression model. The depicted relationship in the multiple regression model between LVEF and age is a relationship with the influence of multiple myocardial infarction "removed". More specifically, we isolated and identified the relationship between LVEF and multiple MI, and isolated and identified the relationship between age and multiple MI, then removed the influence of multiple MI by producing the residuals. Finally, we regressed the residual of LVEF (i.e., what was left of LVEF after removing the multiple MI influence) on the residual of age. So here, by adjusting a relationship, we mean identify, isolate and remove the influences of the adjusting variable. This is done simultaneously in multiple regression analysis by standard software. Thus in the relationship between multiple MI and age in Table 9.3 the influence of age has been isolated, identified, and removed.

So already, we have two sets of p values, one for unadjusted effects, the other for adjusted effects. How do you choose which to use?

Superfits

Since the multiple regression procedure automatically allows for simultaneous adjusting if every independent variable for every other independent variable, a great plethora of findings can and are reported. However, the model from which these findings are reported must be persuasive.

We mentioned earlier in this chapter that one criterion for a model's plausibility is R^2. As we have seen, the greater the sum of squares regression, the better the model's fit to the data. This improved fit has the advantage of increasing the persuasiveness of the model since the model does a good job of explaining the findings in the data. This also reduces the sum of squares error. By reducing this measure of unexplained variability, the power of the test statistic[6] for any of the parameter estimates increases. Thus, a model with a large R^2 has the advantage of greater statistical power. Recognizing this, modern regression software contains tools to automatically build models for a specified dependent variable from a list of candidate independent variables. These procedures work on the principle of maximizing the variability explained by the regression model.

The investigator could increase R^2 by identifying the variables in the dataset that are most "important" himself in the model. However, regression procedures will do this for him automatically. They will search among all candidate variables in the model using established criteria to decide if the inclusion of a particular independent variable will significantly increase R^2. The algorithms are ruthlessly efficient. Some of these work in a forward approach, adding variables one at a time, then choosing the one variable that makes the greatest contribution. Once this has occurred, the system cycles through the remaining independent variables again finding the variable which makes the best contribution to the model, always focused on R^2. Other procedures work backwards, starting with a large model that contains all candidate independent variables, sometimes a hundred or more, then the system searches for the variable that is easiest to drop (i.e., where its loss has the smallest impact on R^2). In this system, the model is "built down" to a smaller collection of variables. Other procedures, termed *stepwise algorithms*, employ a combination of forward and backward examinations. The result is a model that has maximized the variability of the dependent variable that is explained. The more variables, the larger is R^2, the better the fit. The computer "superfits" the model to the data

Thus modern computing facilities permit the creation of automatically generated models in which each included independent variable is statistically significant. The variable selection process, and the simultaneous adjustment of the independent variable-dependent variable relationship for each independent variable are both automatic. This wholesale automation leads to a sense that the researcher is getting something of great value for a very small

---

[6] The concept of power is discussed in chapter 5.

price. Unfortunately, we must remember that the principle *caveat emptor* principle applies—"let the buyer beware".

The difficulty with this fully automated approach is that the purpose of the investigator's analysis has been altered. Such automatically generated models are not built on relationships that are known to exist in the population. To the contrary, they are constructed to maximize the sum of square regression and R^2—and not to maximize the contribution of epidemiology clinical experience, or powers of observation. The blind construction of the model often leads to a result which makes no sense, is uninterpretable, and unacceptable. Plausibility has been sacrificed for statistical power.

This point is worthy of amplification. In general, the dataset will have two classes of relationships, those that are truly representative of the relationships in the population and those are completely spurious, due solely to sampling error. In fact, some relationships that may be present in the population can be absent in the sample. The investigator with a combination of experience in the field and some prospective thought and research will be able to identify these. The automatic variable selection procedures will not—they cannot—differentiate the difference between an association due to sampling error[7] and an association that mirrors a relation that actually resides in the population. Because of the large number of associations these search procedures automatically evaluate, p values are of little help, providing only the coarsest of tools in assessing whether a relationship is real or spurious. This uninterpretability is produced by including independent variables that may have only a transient relationship with the dependent variable in the one dataset—the relationship may be due to sampling error, even with a small p value supporting the argument for the variables' inclusion in the model.

Rather then rest on the bedrock of scientific community experience, these heavyweight models are based only on the shifting sands of sampling error. Thus, variables that are found to be significant can suggest relationships that are completely implausible. Being guided only by levels of significance, these automatic variable selection algorithms yield weak models that often are not

---

[7] An association due to sampling error is an association between a risk factor and an effect in a sample which does not represent the true relationship between the risk factor and the effect in a population.

corroborated by findings from other datasets. This is no surprise, since the model is built on sampling error. Another dataset, drawn at random from the same population, teeming with its own sampling error relationships, will provide a different selection of variables. In variable selection, silicon- based algorithms let us down, and we must rely on our own neurons and intuition to build the model.

Pearls of Great Price

We begin with the acknowledgement that our purpose in carrying out regression analysis is not to report on inconsequential, spurious relationships. Our job is to distill from a database teeming with interrelationships a compact body of knowledge, governed by a few master principles. This requires a thoughtful, deliberate approach.

In my experience, the purpose of most regression analysis is causality argument construction. This purpose often narrows the investigator's focus to a small number of independent variables (principal independent variables) and their relationship with the dependent variable. Generally, these principal independent variables will be related to other variables to which the investigator has access. Other independent variables will also be related to the dependent variables. Let's call the independent variables in which there is no principal interest adjustors. A full review of the literature tempered by discussion with coinvestigators will reveal the identity of these adjustors.

Because of the likelihood of a type I error, adjustors should not be chosen by an automated mechanism. They should be chosen prospectively by the investigator only after considerable thought. Furthermore, if the purpose of the effort is to examine the adjusted relationships between the principal independent variables and the dependent variable, p values for the adjustors should not be provided in the primary analysis, for they will most likely confuse and mislead. The purpose of the regression is not to evaluate the effect of an adjustor and the dependent variable, but to adjust the relationship between the principal independent variable and the dependent variable for the adjustor. The adjusted effects of the principal independent variable are of the greatest important and should be reported.

The more options we have in model building, the more disciplined we must be in using them. Automatic procedures for model building, should be avoided regression analysis in health care because they distract and confuse. Just because we *can* take an action, does not mean we *must* take it. Investigator-generated models stand to contribute the most to the understanding of the elucidated relationship. Since adjustors were chosen from the literature, they have some basis other than sampling error for inclusion in the model — they have scientific community support. In addition, other researchers with experience in the field know from the literature the potential importance of the adjustors, and will expect them in the analysis. An automatic (silicon-based) approach will use tens and sometimes hundreds of p values to build a model that rests on only the thin reed of sampling error. The investigator-based (neuron) model rests on strength of evidence from the literature and the scientific community, and uses only a small number of p values to provide an assessment of the statistical significance of the relationships between the principal independent variables and the dependent variable. Being they are easy to interpret and incorporate into scientific communities fund of knowledge, such models are pearls of great price.

Effect Modifiers and Alpha Allocation

We have seen that a disciplined approach to model construction in regression analysis can allow an investigator to report on the effects of principal independent variables. These effects are reported after adjusting for (i.e., isolating, identifying, and removing) the influences of adjustors. However, regression analysis is not limited to these direct or main effects. Regression analysis can also report interaction effects, or effect modifiers. Interaction terms exerts their influence by modifying the relationship between a principal independent variable and the dependent variable. They are elegant, but complicated. P value interpretation for these effects must be approached with great care.

Interactive Models
Thus far, we have used the three Hill criteria of plausibility consistency, and coherency in the regression model building process.

Interpretability of the model is often enhanced with the explicit consideration of interactive terms.

Consider the database the investigator has been interrogating thus far, with particular attention to differentiating myocardial infarction location. There are two dichotomous variables for the three myocardial infarction locations: anterior lateral, posterior, and inferior. The investigator defines dichotomous variables x_1 ($= 1$ if the heart attack is posterior, 0 otherwise) and x_2 ($= 1$ if the heart attack occurs inferiorly, 0 otherwise). Consider the following model.

$$E[y_i] = \beta_0 + \beta_1 x_{1i} + \beta_2 x_{2i} + \beta_3 age + \beta_4 x_{1i} age + \beta_5 x_{2i} age.$$

Note the last two terms in the model, which are product terms. Let's examine this model and its implications carefully. For a patient who has an anterolateral myocardial infarction

$$E[y_i] = \beta_0 + \beta_3 age.$$

This model states that ejection fraction is a function of age (and an intercept). For a patient of the same age with a posterior MI.

$$E[y_i] = \beta_0 + \beta_1 x_{1i} + \beta_3 age + \beta_4 x_{1i} age ,$$

which can be rewritten as

$$E[y_i] = (\beta_0 + \beta_1) + (\beta_3 + \beta_4) age .$$

This reflects an important change from the model relating LVEF to age for patients with an anterolateral heart attack. Note that in patients with a posterior myocardial infarction, this model depicts a straightline relationship between LVEF and age, but a different relationship from the one identified for patients with an anterolateral heart attack.. The relationship for patients with a posterior MI has a different intercept (not just β_1, but $\beta_1 + \beta_2$) and a different slope (not just β_3, but $\beta_3 + \beta_4$). β_4 is of particular interest, since it represents the way MI location affects the relationship between LVEF and age. We have a similar implication for patients with a myocardial infarction located inferiorly, specified by the model

$$E[y_i] = (\beta_0 + \beta_2) + (\beta_3 + \beta_5) age$$

The interpretations of these models lead directly to some interesting hypotheses. One interesting hypothesis is whether there is any impact of infarct location on LVEF. Examining these models, we see that infarct location can have multiple effects on LVEF, through of β_1, β_2, β_4, or β_5. or any combination

Effect Modifiers can be Difficult to Explain.

Interaction terms in regression models can be very attractive, but the effects they measure can be complicated to explain. The relationship between the principal independent variable age and left ventricular ejection fraction is straightforward. As we have seen earlier in this chapter, older patients tend to have lower ejection fractions than younger patients. However, the inclusion of the product term suggests that this relationship between age and LVEF is a function of a heart attack's location. This is a much more complicated relationship for the medical community to absorb. The investigator should be sure that this relationship is not likely to be due to sampling error, and should have carefully considered a priori evidence for including the term before accepting the effect modifying influence of myocardial infarction location.

Unfortunately, this is not often the case. The current feeling is that significance levels for effect sizes (i.e., p values) to be included in the model should be on the order of 0.10 or even larger. This is often motivated by the understandable desire to avoid ignoring an important new effect—i.e., the investigators don't want to miss anything, Unfortunately, what they catch is sampling error. In addition, interaction terms can be very difficult to explain to practitioners. Main effects are direct, easily understood, while interaction terms are complex. Trying to explain a complicated interaction term based on a weak finding at a level of significance of 0.10 or higher is often only a futile attempt to explain shifting patterns in the sampling error sands.

As an alternative approach, consider the following cross sectional evaluation. An investigator has obtained demographic and lipid data on 4,159 patients who have sustained a heart attack. He is interested in identifying demographic measures that may be related to LDL cholesterol levels. He will do this using a cross-sectional design[8]. Before his evaluation begins, he does a thor-

---

[8] The strengths and weaknesses of cross-sectional designs were discussed in chapter three.

Table 9.5. Prospective Alpha Allocation for Predictors of LDL

Effect	Allocated Alpha
Interactions	
Age—gender interaction	0.003
Exercise-gender interaction	0.003
All other externally suggested interactions	0.003
Main Effects	
Age	0.024
Gender	0.040
Race	0.040
Family History of CVD	0.040
Country	0.040
Smoking	0.024
Alcohol	0.024
Exercise	0.024
Diabetes	0.024
Hypertension	0.024
Beta blocker use	0.024

ough literature review and consults with other lipid specialists. His review of the literature strongly suggests that each of the main effects of age, gender, race, country, and family history of heart disease are related to LDL cholesterol levels. The investigator also notes that others have suggested that each of smoking history, alcohol consumption, exercise level diabetes, hypertension, and beta blockers use may exert influence as well, although the evidence for these latter variables is somewhat weaker. In addition, the investigator's own assimilation of the available information suggests that several interactions may be of interest. One is that age may influence the relationship between gender and baseline LDL cholesterol (i.e., there is a significant age gender interaction). A second interaction of interest is exercise and gender. He has also been convinced by other investigators that several other interactions about which he has no strong feeling may be present.

The investigator must consider his decision strategy and alpha allocation decisions carefully. He believes a priori that the previously mentioned interactions may be present, but he understands the difficulty of arguing persuasively for them, since a relationship modifying effect is more difficult to explain than a main effect. For example, explaining that the effect of exercise on LDL cholesterol levels is related to gender, and that women may have to exercise more than men, is a complicated message to deliver to a scientific community that is already overwhelmed by advice on reducing risk factors for heart disease. Similarly, patients are often confused by complex messages from the health community. The investigator recognizes this, and responds that he will argue for an interaction effect only if its "signal" is strong enough. If the alpha error is too great, he is unwilling to attempt to make a persuasive argument for an effect size. He chooses to apportion type I error as described in Table 9.5.

The investigator apportions 0.003 alpha to each interaction of interest, and an additional 0.003 to the group of interactions suggested by others. For the main effects, he allocates 0.04 each to gender, race, country and family history of heart disease, with 0.024 for the other main effects. The results are as follows.

This table shows the interaction effects first, since main effects cannot be assessed in the presence of interactions. Since none of the interactions met the criteria of significance, and they all may now be removed from the model. The remainder of table displays the unadjusted and adjusted effects of the candidate risk factors on LDL cholesterol levels. Z scores and p values are shown only for the adjusted effects, because none of the characteristics were assigned randomly, and attribution of effect size will be easily confounded among these correlated main effects. The results may be summarized as follows.

In exploratory evaluations of baseline LDL cholesterol correlates, no model explained more than 1.5 percent of the total variability of LDL cholesterol. No interaction term made a significant contribution to the ability of any covariate to explain LDL cholesterol variability. Gender and diabetes each provided significant reductions in unexplained LDL cholesterol variability. Women had a 0.05 mg/dl lower LDL cholesterol than men, after adjusting for age, race, history of atherosclerotic cardiovascular disease, country, smoking, alcohol, exercise, diabetes, hypertension, and beta blockers($p = 0.020$). Diabetics had a 0.08 mg/dl lower baseline LDL cholesterol than nondiabetics, after adjustment ($P < 0.001$).

Conclusion

Regression analysis provides a powerful tool for exploring the relationships between potentially influential factors and dependent

Table 9.6. Results of Baseline LDL Evaluation

Total Alpha	0.30
Alpha for Interaction	0.01
Alpha for main effects	0.29

Interactions	Allocated Alpha	P value	Conclusion
Age group	0.003	>0.5	Insignificant
Exercise group	0.003	>0.5	Insignificant
Others	0.003	>0.5	Insignificant

Main Effects

Variable	Allocated Alpha	Unadjusted		Adjusted			Conclusions
		Effect Size	Std Error of Effect Size	Effect Size	Std Error of Effect Size	P	
Age	0.024	-0.068	0.024	-0.002	0.001	0.027	Insignificant
Gender	0.040	-1.254	0.654	-0.050	0.026	0.020	Significant
Race	0.040	1.278	0.863	0.051	0.035	0.543	Insignificant
Family History	0.040	0.168	0.461	0.007	0.018	0.090	Insignificant
Country	0.024	-1.250	0.477	-0.030	0.011	0.090	Insignificant
Smoking	0.024	1.115	0.614	0.027	0.015	0.325	Insignificant
Alcohol	0.024	0.236	0.492	0.006	0.012	0.638	Insignificant
Exercise	0.024	0.795	0.457	0.019	0.011	0.028	Insignificant
Diabetes	0.024	-3.361	0.647	-0.081	0.016	<0.001	Significant
Hypertension	0.024	-0.560	0.457	-0.013	0.011	0.241	Insignificant
Beta Blockers	0.024	-0.631	0.462	-0.015	0.011	0.699	Insignificant

variables. However, the careful investigator must be sensitive to the extent to which he turns control of the analysis over to the computer. Computers can provide important useful information, such as effect size and variance estimates. However, the investigator should wrest control of variable selection from automatic search procedures, which work to build maximum R^2 models. Since population based relationships as well as sampling error based relationships are embedded in the analysis sample, the investigator needs a tool to differentiate these influences. The best tool is not the computer, which will not distinguish these sources of relationships, but the investigator himself. By diligently reviewing the literature, the investigator is in the best position to distinquish the real relationships from the spurious ones. If the idea is to go on a fishing expedition for significance, what is caught is often only the junk of sampling error.

Alpha allocation plays an important role in interpreting regression analyses. Effect modification influences should be carefully considered before the analysis is undertaken. If the purpose of the experiment is to tease out an interaction effect, the investigator may justifiably increase alpha. However, if the interactions are not expected, then their biologic nonplausibility and tangled explanations argue for a small type I error level. Finally, by understanding the role of adjustment (identification, isolation, and removal of the adjustor's effects) in regression analysis, the investigator can usefully disentangle confounded effects. However, the lack of the use of randomization tightly circumscribes the contribution such regression models can make to causality arguments.

Finally consider the stethoscope. It is a well designed, finely tuned tool for physicians and others to interpret informative body sounds. Yet, despite its craftsmanship, the most important part of this instrument is the part between our ears. The most important component of computer based regression analyses is the same.

10

CHAPTER

Bayesian *P* Values

There are no substitutes for *p* values when a statistical interrogation must lead to a decision. It will therefore come as no surprise when I say that their use requires careful, deliberate thought. Even in the simplest of experiments, investigators must think critically and prospectively about the degree of community protection they wish to provide as they determine the type I and type II errors. As I pointed out in chapters 7 and 8, the application of *p* values to experiments in health care is even more complicated when these experiments have more than two treatment arms and multiple endpoints. In all cases, the experiment must be executed concordantly, according to the protocol, so that the resulting *p* values are interpretable. These endeavors are not to be undertaken lightly.

But what an arbitrary process! The best, most community-oriented physician-scientist who possesses firm knowledge of the possible efficacy and side effects of the compound to be studied, must eventually, finally settle on alpha levels for each of the experiment's endpoints. How does he finally decide on 0.17 for one endpoint, 0.083 for another, and 0.035 for a third? What precisely is the reasoning process? The investigator thinks carefully, but in the end, he settles on a choice. The arbitrary nature of the choice and the absence of firm rules for the selection (apart from the knee-jerk 0.05 choice which requires no thought at all) is a singular handicap of this process. The choice would be less problematic if there were some direct rules one could follow that responded to

234

the properties of the intervention and the unique features of the subject population being studied. However, there are no such rules.

It is no wonder that practitioners are flummoxed by this selection process.[1] Alpha allocation reflects a thought process very different from the customary thinking of physicians in clinical practice. In fact, we must acknowledge that, by and large, practicing physicians are left out of the construction aspect of research. Practitioners are seen not as contributors to, but as consumers of large clinical research programs. Earlier[2] we pointed out that the nature of the practitioner's focus on individual patients limits that practitioner's ability to objectively discern the benefits and hazards of a particular intervention. They must embrace the tools of population sampling and well-designed intervention testing experiments in order to gain this objectivity.

However, although we have suggested that these physicians embrace the results of well-designed experiments, we have said nothing about the possible contributions they could make. Of course, clinical trials do use these practitioners' patients, working hard to randomize those who meet the trial entry criteria to their studies, while guaranteeing that the clinical trial would not completely take the patient away from the practitioner. This patient contribution must not be minimized, for if the trial results are to be generalizable, the trial must include patients who are representative of the population. This contribution by practicing physicians is invaluable. Also, the clinician provides strategies on how to help patients stay on the study medication, and comply with their follow-up visits. However, we know that the concepts of community protection, the tools used by physician scientists in designing trials, are very different from the tools used by practitioners in their day-to-day treatment of individual patients. Is this difference so great that it precludes any intellectual contribution by practitioners to well-designed trials? Is there no room for the possibility that these practitioners may be able to contribute at a more central level, providing insight into event rates of disease and the degree to which the intervention may be effective? Does their experience count for nothing in the research process, beyond ignition of the initial idea and the valuable contribution of their patients?

In general, clinical trials accept practitioners' patients, leaving

---

[1] Dr. Kassell's reaction in the introduction is a fine example here.
[2] See chapter 1.

these doctors and nurses limited opportunity to contribute to the experiment's construction. Those who design these experiments are part of small shop of "super investigators," biostatisticians, epidemiologists, and administrators. To be sure, their special expertise is required, and incorporation of multitudinous, disparate information from private practitioners' experiences for event rate construction would be intractable within the traditionally accepted significance testing paradigm. However, the trial built only on the expertise of the designers, without due consideration of the experience of the practitioners who have been seeing these patients for years before the trial's inception, is at best squandering a useful resource, and perhaps is also perhaps somewhat unrepresentative. Can we expect practitioners to embrace an experiment's results if they have been excluded from the research construction? Is there no way to inject a practitioner's intellectual contribution into the clinical trial cognitive repository?

Recently, there has been a good deal of discussion about the Bayesian approach to statistical reasoning. The Bayes philosophy appears to place less pre-experimental emphasis on the type I error, in favor of posterior *p* values. In addition, its required stipulation of loss functions and prior distributions provides for the broad input of the many and not the narrow digested input of a few. The Bayes approach is designed specifically to accept diverse experiences of contributors, building up a formal integrated view of this knowledge. This concept is new and novel to statistical reasoning in research medicine and requires some attention.

The Bayesian approach to statistics is a diverse and growing field. Like grass in the spring (some would say like weeds), it is pushing up into all branches of statistics, providing a fresh perspective on estimation and hypothesis testing in statistics. In this chapter, we will discuss the difference between classical and Bayesian statistics, explain the new features offered by Bayesian statistics, and provide an example of the use of Bayesian statistics in a hypothesis testing situation. However, we must note that, just as for the classical approach, the correct use of Bayes procedures requires disciplined, prospective thought.

The Frequentists vs. the Bayesians

The Bayesian approach disturb classical statisticians just as malpractice issues affects physicians—these issues both produce not only cerebral responses, but emotional anguish as well. The computational underpinnings of Bayes procedures rely on the straightforward application of well-established conditional probability theory. However, the philosophical foundation of the Bayes approach with its frank and explicit use of prior information and its invocation of loss functions, is often the subject of heated controversy. Let's take just a moment to view classical statistics (practiced by "frequentists") before we turn attention to Bayesian statistics as practiced by "Bayesians."

Classical statistics is the collection of statistical techniques and devices that evaluate the accuracy of a technique in terms of its long-term repetitive accuracy [1]. Significance testing is a familiar example of this approach. It may not provide the correct solution for an individual experiment. Its virtue is in its long-term accuracy. Several prices are paid for this. The first is the interesting construction of significance testing. We never reject the null hypothesis, we just refuse to accept it. We never accept the alternative hypothesis—we reject the null hypothesis. In fact, the null hypothesis was so called by Fisher because it was the hypothesis to be nullified by the data. The entire formulation of the hypothesis testing paradigm to nonstatisticians appears backward. They would like to know the probability that their idea is correct, not the reverse probability that the idea they do not believe is incorrect. To many workers in health care, the mathematics of statistics is complicated enough without engaging in this awkward, serpentine reasoning process.

Another problem of classical statistics is its concentration not just on what has occurred, but also on what has *not* occurred in a research program. How these nonoccurrences are handled can have a dramatic impact on the answer to the hypothesis test, and preoccupation with them can bedevil the result interpreter. Consider the following example, adapted from Lindley [2]. A physician who staffs a cardiology clinic believes that more than half of his patients have hypertension. He is interested in carrying out an observational study to test this hypothesis. The cardiologist proceeds by keeping track of the patients who come into the clinic. He decides to count how many patients he must see until there are three who do not have hypertension. If hypertension is as prevalent as he suspects, this count will be high. On this particular morning, he saw twelve patients ($n = 12$) until three did not have hypertension ($y = 3$). These results reveal a prevalence of 75 percent. Emboldened by these findings, which he believes are strong enough to represent a statement about the prevalence of hypertension in the population, he consults a statistician. The cardiologist explains the rationale and method for the research, and provides his findings. He asks the statistician to construct a *p* value for this program. After hearing how the study was executed, the statistician begins:

$$p \text{ value} = \text{Prob [test statistic falls in the critical region} \\ \text{when the null hypothesis is true]}$$

$$P[n = 12, y = 3] + P[n = 13, y = 3] + P[n = 14, y = 3] \\ + P[n = 15, y = 3] + P[n = 16, y = 3] + P[n = 17, y = 3] + \cdots$$

The cardiologist is perplexed. Why are all of these terms necessary? He understands why the first term, $P[n = 12, y = 3]$, has to be included, since it represents the data that was observed. But what about these other terms, $P[n = 13, y = 3]$, $P[n = 14, y = 3]$, etc.? He did not observe thirteen or fourteen patients, only twelve. He does not want to misrepresent his argument, so why include probabilities for events that did not take place? The statistician replies that the *p* value construction was based not only on the results as they occurred but also on results that are more extreme. The statistician then turns back to compute the sum of these probabilities, which is 0.0325. The *p* value is 0.0325, a small number, suggesting to the cardiologist that, in the population from which he sees patients, hypertension is indeed prevalent. The cardiologist, although pleased with the outcome, nevertheless harbors some suspicion about the inclusive nature of these computations, and is concerned about this practice of including "results" in the computation that did not occur in the research effort. Since he is in the clinic the next day, the cardiologist decides to carry out another observational study, and consult another statistician.

The next day, he chooses to observe his clinic for a specified period, counting the patients who attend the clinic, and tabulating the number with hypertension. The cardiologist observes that twelve patients have appeared in clinic, nine of whom have high blood pressure. This is again a prevalence of 0.75. The consistency of these results bolsters the cardiologist's confidence that the occurrence of hypertension is indeed high. Taking his results to a second statistician, he watches as she begins. She starts with letting θ be the prevalence of hypertension in this population. Then she finds

$$P \text{ value} = \text{Prob [test statistic falls in the critical region}$$
$$\text{when the null hypothesis is true]}$$

$$= P[x = 9|\theta = 1/2] + P[x = 10|\theta = 1/2]$$
$$+ P[x = 11|\theta = 1/2] + P[x = 12|\theta = 1/2].$$

Again, the cardiologist is vexed. This statistician, like the other, starts with the observed result (nine patients with hypertension out of twelve patients seen), but continues by considering more extreme findings). This time however, the cardiologist is shocked to find that the sum of these probabilities is 0.075, much greater than the 0.0325 produced by the first statistician. Not only has the same data generated different results, but the results are very much dependent on events that did not occur. In fact, the issue is somewhat worse. Under the null hypothesis, these nonoccurring, extreme events were very unlikely anyway. So, the p value is dependent not only on events that did not occur, but it is dependent on events that would not have been expected to occur. To many non-statisticians constructing a decision rule based on the non-occurrence of unlikely events appears nonsensical.

This cardiologist bemoans his problem to an internist, who describes the following experience in her own clinic (adapted from Pratt [3]).

"I was just interested in producing a confidence interval for diastolic blood pressures in my clinic. That's all I wanted to do. I had an automated device that would read blood pressure very accurately and produce data that appeared to be normally distributed with a mean of 87 and a standard deviation of 5. After collecting this data, I turned it over to a statistician who carried out the simple analysis. When the statistician came to my clinic to share his findings, he fell into a conversation with the staff nurse who told him that the automated blood-pressure-measuring device did not read above 100 mm Hg. When I confirmed this, the statistician said that he now had to do a new analysis, removing the underlying assumption of normality since the blood pressure cuff would read any diastolic blood pressures greater than 100 mm Hg as 100 mm Hg, thus violating the assumption of a normal distribution. I understood his point, but assured him that in my data, no patient had a diastolic blood pressure greater than 97 mm Hg, and if it had been, I would have called another clinic for a backup automated device equally sensitive to BP readings greater than 100 mm Hg. The statistician was relieved, thanked me, and returned to his office. However, after he left, I noticed that my backup unit was broken, and e-mailed him about this. He e-mailed me back saying that he would have to redo the analysis after all! I was astonished and called him immediately. Why should the analysis be redone? No blood pressure was greater than 100 mm Hg, so the broken backup device would not have had to be used. My measurements were just as precise and accurate as they would have been if all instruments were working fine. The results would have been no different. Soon he would be asking me about my stethoscope!"

The Bayesian Philosophy

These amusing anecdotes demonstrates how classical statisticians base their analyses on what did not occur, and the understandable befuddlement of those they work with. The Bayesian formulation, on the other hand, is based in the likelihood principle, which states that a decision should have its foundation in what has occurred, not in what has not occurred. Like classical statistics, Bayes theory is applicable to problems of parameter estimation and hypothesis testing. Before turning to hypothesis testing, we will spend just a moment discussing Bayesian parameter estimation since the underlying formulation is the same.

The problem of Bayes estimation can be stated as attempting to estimate the population parameter θ of a distribution (just as frequentists do). The Bayes estimation process requires the analyst to be specific about the probability distribution for the data and the distribution for θ as well, and also to make a clear statement about loss functions. Bayes theory works forward from conditional probability theory, identifying the distribution of θ given the data that has been observed. This is a different viewpoint than that taken by the frequentists which assumes the parameter θ is a constant. From the Bayes perspective, θ has its own distribution called the prior distribution $\Pi(\theta)$. This prior distribution reflects knowledge about the location and behavior of θ before the experiment is carried out. After the experiment is executed, we have new information, which is combined with the prior information to obtain a new estimate of θ. This is accomplished by combining the data x whose conditional distribution with respect to θ is known $f_x(x|\theta)$. The statistician will then compute the posterior distribution of θ given x $(\Pi_\theta(\theta|x))$ as

$$\Pi(\theta|x) = \frac{f_x(x|\theta)\ \Pi(\theta)}{\int_{\Omega_\theta} f_x(x|\theta)\ \Pi(\theta)} \qquad (10.1)$$

This looks complicated, and, in fact, it usually is . Fortunately, we do not have to bother about the details of this computation. The point is that information concerning the parameter of interest, θ, goes through a series of stages. With no observation from which to work, our best information for θ comes from $\Pi(\theta)$, the prior distribution of θ. After x is observed, we combine the information learned about θ from the research with the information known about θ obtained from $\Pi(\theta)$, and assemble the posterior distribution of θ. In this way, the posterior distribution contains information from prior knowledge of θ and information gathered from observing the data.

Prior Distributions
Before we can proceed, we must ask ourselves, does a prior distribution make sense? The concept that the population parameter has its own variability stands in stark contrast to the perspective of the classical (frequentist) approach, in which no consideration is given and no allowance made for variability in population parameters. The only source of variability the frequentists consider is sampling variability (the variability that comes from the sample). Consider blood glucose measurements. If we apply comments about sampling schemes from chapter 1, we would say that if the investigator could measure everybody's blood glucose everywhere, he would have determined the blood glucose measurement exactly. However, this admittedly impossible task may itself be something of a simplification. The blood glucose measurement for an individual is not a constant but a quantity that varies. It changes with time of day, activity level digestive state, hormonal status, etc. Certainly, this intrinsic, biologic variability is better approximated by applying a probability distribution to it, and not assuming it is a fixed, unmovable target. The incorporation of a prior distribution is one of the hallmarks of a Bayesian analysis.

The Loss Function
A second feature of Bayesian analysis is the sense of loss. The end of the Bayesian computation is not the determination of the posterior distribution. The Bayesian must decide what to do with that distribution. What they do with it depends on the loss function they use. The loss function determines what loss the user sustains when they attempt to take an action. That action may be to identify an estimator for the parameter θ, or it may be to make a decision about the location of θ (i.e., decide that $\theta = 0$). The Bayesian con-

structs the loss function to reflect the true consequences of correct and incorrect decisions. Once the loss function is defined, it tells the investigator how to use the posterior distribution to take an action. The loss function is denoted as $L(\theta, \delta)$, where θ is the parameter to be estimated and δ is the estimator to be used.

For example, if the purpose of the analysis is to estimate cholesterol levels, a common loss function to use is squared error loss $L(\theta, \delta) = (\theta - \delta)^2$. This error is the smallest of course when $\theta = \delta$, i.e., when the estimate is equal to the parameter. However, it also says that the further the estimator δ is from the parameter θ (i.e., the worse our estimate is), the loss we incur increases, and increases quadratically. Another implication of this loss function is that the penalty is the same for underestimating θ as for overestimating θ.

The Bayesian estimator is the quantity that minimizes the average loss. This averaging is taken over the updated information for θ, i.e., from the posterior distribution. Thus, the loss function is used in combination with the posterior density to identify the estimator which reduces the expected values of the loss function or the risk. If the loss function is squared error loss, the Bayes estimator δ is the mean of the posterior distribution. If the loss function is absolute error loss, then the Bayes estimator is the median of the posterior distribution. Thus the loss function determines how the posterior density is to be used to find δ.

Example of Bayesian Estimation

For example, let's assume that the prior probability distribution of total cholesterol follows a normal distribution with mean μ and variance τ^2. The investigator wishes to update this information for the mean cholesterol value; he collects a random sample of individuals from the population, measuring their cholesterol values. He assumes that the cholesterol values obtained from his sample follow a normal distribution as well, but with mean θ and variance σ^2. If the investigator were to use the frequentist approach, he would simply estimate θ, the mean cholesterol value by the sample mean of his data. Although there is variability associated with this estimate (σ^2/n), it is important to note that this variability is associated with only the sampling scheme i.e., variability associated with the sample mean, not the population mean. The population mean is seen as fixed. The sample mean, because of sampling error, contains all of the variability.

However, the Bayesian doesn't just take the mean cholesterol level of his sample, he combines his data with the prior distribution to construct the posterior distribution. In this case when the prior distribution is normal with mean μ: and variance τ^2 and the conditional distribution is normal with mean θ and variance σ^2, the posterior distribution of θ given x is also normal. The mean of this posterior distribution, $\Pi(\theta|x)$ is

$$\mu_p = \frac{\tau^2}{\sigma^2/dn + \tau^2}\bar{x} + \frac{\sigma^2/n}{\sigma^2/n + \tau^2}\mu$$

and variance v_p^2

$$v_p = (n/\sigma^2 + 1/\tau^2)^{-1}$$

Let's take a moment to examine these quantities. The posterior mean μ_p depends not just on the distribution of x, but also depends on the parameters μ and τ^2 from the prior distribution as well. The posterior mean is a weighted average of the mean of the prior distribution and the sample mean obtained from the data. The prior mean μ has been updated to the posterior mean μ_p by the sample data. Similarly, the prior variance τ^2 has been updated to the posterior variance $v_p{}^2$ by the incorporation of σ^2. If we are using squared error loss the Bayes estimate δ_β of the parameter θ, then

$$\delta_\beta = \frac{\tau^2}{\sigma^2/n + \tau^2}\bar{x} + \frac{\sigma^2/n}{\sigma^2/n + \tau^2}\mu$$

Bayesian *P* values

Significance testing is easily within the Bayesians' reach. In earlier chapters we have argued for the arbitrary choice of type I and type II errors. We have argued that they should be chosen prospectively, we have argued that they should be chosen thoughtfully, but we have always argued that they should be chosen. The Bayesian approach is not so preoccupied with the arbitrary choice of alpha levels. However, there must be prospective interpretation of other quantities.

In the classical approach, we are concerned with making a decision about an unknown parameter θ (e.g. the mean of a distribution, or a cumulative incidence rate). We obtain a collection of observations from the population. This collection of observations has a probability distribution which depends on θ. Since the probability distribution of the data depends on θ, each observation in the data containing some information about θ. Thus, in estimation, we find a function of the x's which allows us to estimate θ. In significance testing, we identify a function of the x's which allow us to make a decision about θ (e.g. $\theta = 0.25$ vs. $\theta \neq 0.25$).

The Bayesian approach uses probability distributions as well. Like the classical formulation, it is concerned with the probability distribution of the collection of x's when θ is known (called $f(x|\theta)$). However, as we have seen, the Bayesian view is that θ itself is not fixed, but has a probability distribution based on other parameters. This distribution is called the prior distribution (i.e., it is known prior to collecting data). Bayesians will combine this prior distribution of θ with the conditional distribution of x given θ to obtain the posterior distribution θ given x. This can be usefully viewed as a process of updating information. Before the experiment begins, something is known about θ, although its exact value remains unknown. For example, in a research effort that will estimate cumulative mortality in a population, the investigator knows that the cumulative mortality rate is between 0.20 and 0.30. He may not be sure of its exact value, but previous work has placed it in this region. The investigator then collects a random collection of subjects from the population and observes the death rate in this sample. These data provide information about θ, since they follow the conditional distribution $f(x|\theta)$. The investigator then computes the posterior distribution of θ given x. This procedure updates the information about θ from the prior distribution to the posterior distribution. The loss function tells the Bayesian how to use the posterior distribution to carry out the evaluation.

Example of Bayes Hypothesis Testing: Asthma Prevalence in a Clinic

Classical statisticians talk about significance testing. Bayesians talk about taking *action*. In hypothesis testing, the Bayesian acts, taking an action to either accept or reject a hypothesis. However, like with frequentists, they must *think* before they act.

Consider the example of a clinic whose administrator needs to decide whether the proportion of patients it sees with asthma is greater than 5 percent during the summer months. If the proportion is larger, the clinic administrator will need to invest resources in the clinic to so that it may better serve its community. This will involve both an education program for the clinic staff and the provision of ample medical supplies to treat asthma. In his quest to determine the proportion of asthma patients seen in the summer months, the administrator approaches the clinic doctors, and learns that they are not at all sure of the prevalence of this problem in their patients. They do agree that its prevalence is greater than 1 percent and less than 20 percent, but can reach no consensus on a more refined estimate. Let's watch the administrator take a Bayesian action.

Let θ be the prevalence of asthma. In order to take a Bayesian action in this problem of testing for the location of θ, the administrator must be armed with

1 the prior distribution of θ,
2 the distribution of the data obtained in his sample, and
3 the loss function

He uses the information provided by the physicians is used to estimate the prior distribution of θ. If no one value in this range of 0.01 to 0.20 is more likely than any other, he can spread the prior probability uniformly over this region[3]. He can also identify the distribution of the estimated proportion of patients with asthma from a sample of clinic data. If the number of patients who visit the clinic is n, then the prevalence of asthma patients follows a normal distribution with mean θ and variance $\theta(1 - \theta)/n$[4].

Having identified the prior distribution of θ and the distribution of the data from the sample, the administrator now must consider the loss function. He begins by considering the two possible actions he can take. Let the first action (a_1) be the decision that $\theta < 0.05$. Let the second action (a_2) the decision that $\theta \geq 0.05$. The

---

[3] Some critics would argue that assuming probability is equally distributed across this region is assuming knowledge about the location of θ . Here we use it to provide an example, not to justify the approach.

[4] This is just saying that the probability of the number of asthma cases in a sample of n patients when θ is known follows the binomial distribution.

Table 10.1. Loss function for Asthma Proportion Decision

		Possible Actions	
		a_1 (decide $\theta < 0.05$)	a_2 (decide $\theta \geq 0.05$)
Location of θ	$\theta < 0.05$	0	cost $k_2 = \$1500$
	$\theta \geq 0.05$	cost $k_1 = \$10,000$	0

administrator can make one and only one decision about the location of θ, and recognizes that that decision will be either right or wrong. Let's say the administrator takes action a_1, deciding that $\theta < 0.05$. If he is right then he incurs no loss. However he is wrong then the clinic will incur a cost. That cost is not being prepared for the asthma patients that will visit the clinic. This means lost patients to the clinic and some diminution of the clinic's reputation in the community. The administrator denotes this cost by k_1, setting $k_1 = \$10,000$.

Now, the administrator could take action a_2, deciding that θ is greater than 0.05. Again, he could be right or wrong. If he is correct, the cost is zero. If he is wrong, then he has has invested more money into the clinic staff training and supplies than was necessary. Call that cost k_2, and set $k_2 = \$1500$. The loss function could be represented as a Table 10.1

The Bayesian action is the action which produces the smallest loss. To determine what action the administrator should take, he computes his average loss E_p for each possible decision. If he takes action a_1 his loss is

$$E_P[L(\theta, a_1)] = L(\theta < 0.05, a_1)P[\theta < 0.05] + L(\theta \geq 0.05, a_1)P[\theta \geq 0.05]$$
$$= k_1 P[\theta \geq 0.05]$$

If the administrator takes action a_2 he incurs the following average loss.

$$E_P[L(\theta, a_2)] = L(\theta < 0.05, a_2)P[\theta < 0.05] + L(\theta \geq 0.05, a_2)P[\theta \geq 0.05]$$
$$= k_2 P[\theta < 0.05].$$

The administrator chooses action a_2 when its expected or average loss for action a_2 is less than that expected loss for action a_1. Note this average loss is averaged over the values of θ (i.e., its probability distribution). This means that the administrator must know the distribution of θ. He already knows the prior distribution of θ, so what he now requires is the posterior distribution of θ. Thus, the administrator chooses action a_2 when

$$k_1 P[\theta \geq 0.05] > k_2 P[\theta < 0.05].$$

Now if we let $p = P[\theta \geq 0.05]$, we see that $1 - p = P[\theta < 0.05]$. The application of some algebra reveals that the administrator should

$$decide\ \theta \geq 0.05\ if\ \ p > \frac{k_2}{k_1 + k_2}$$

where $p = P[\theta \geq 0.05]$. This is the decision rule. The administrator's choices $k_1 = \$10,000$, $k_2 = \$1500$ lead to the decision rule to decide in favor of $\theta \geq 0.05$, if p is greater than 0.1304.

The administrator needs to identify the distribution of θ to choose the Bayes action. He already has the distribution of θ based on the prior distribution; the beliefs of the clinic physicians suggested that the proportion of asthma cases was between 1 percent and 20 percent. However, he cannot base his judgment solely on their beliefs, since these beliefs are based on their own experiences and are subject to bias and distortion. He assesses the proportion of patients identified in the clinic during the past summer, and finds that this proportion is 0.065. The administrator can now compute (or have computed for him) the $p\ [\theta \geq 0.05]$, using the posterior probability distribution. For our problem the mathematics lead to

$$p = \frac{\int_{0.05}^{0.20} \sqrt{\dfrac{n}{2\pi(1-\theta)}}\, e^{-(n(\theta-x)^2/2\theta(1-\theta))}\, d\theta}{\int_{0.01}^{0.20} \sqrt{\dfrac{n}{2\pi\theta(1-\theta)}}\, e^{-(n(\theta-x)^2/2\theta(1-\theta))}\, d\theta} \qquad (10.2)$$

which is the ratio of two normal probabilities. Using the value $x = 0.065$ in 10.2 he computes that $p = 0.929$. Since this quantity is greater than 0.1304, he concludes that θ is greater than 0.05, and proceeds with the additional training and supply procurement.

It might be useful to consider the implications of this rule. Let's see how this rule changes based on the value of x. If x were 0.050, $P(\theta \geq 0.05) = 0.541$, the decision would have been to expand the asthma service. If $x = 0.040$, $P(\theta \geq 0.05) = 0.209$ and the decision would have again been to expand the asthma service. Only when $x < 0.036$ would the decision have been to keep the asthma service unchanged. How could this be? If $x < 0.05$, why is the $P(\theta \geq 0.05)$ still high? The answer resides in the loss function.

This function is built on the premise that the worst error would be not to expand the services when they should be expanded. This is transmitted directly to the decision rule, which pushes for expansion even with asthma prevalence values of 0.04.

Note that this exercise in stating a problem, drawing a sample, and making a decision based on that sample was carried out without a single statement about significance testing or type I or type II error. The administrator computed a single posterior probability. However, this probability has the look and feel of a *p* value even it is not derived from a classical hypothesis test. It is based on a loss function, which is new to frequentists. However, the identifications of the table entries in Table 10.1 seemed suspiciously like the thought process involved in deciding on the values of type I and type II error. However, the paradigm was different. In this case, he did not have tradition to guide (or misguide) him. He simply estimated the costs of the possible mistakes he could make, then followed a procedure to minimize these costs. The decisions he had to make were analogous to those made for *p* value computation, but they were asked in more concrete terms and in where in which he could provide direct answers.

Also note that administrator could have taken the approach of going only by the physician beliefs, i.e., the prior distribution. This would have been a mistake, since, as pointed out in chapter 1, the focus of practicing physician's on the patient distorts their perception of the true proportion of events. It is easy and correct to justify the need for a more objective measurement of the proportion of patients with asthma by taking a sample of data from the clinic.

However, we must examine the other side of this coin. Once the administrator has collected his sample of data and obtained a sample estimate of 0.065 for the proportion of patients with asthma, why not just discard the physician opinions? In fact, if the administrator had consulted a frequentist statistician, this is precisely what would have happened. The frequentist would have constructed a binomial test of proportions covered in an elementary statistics course and carry out a straightforward hypothesis test, using only the data and discarding the physician beliefs.

By sticking with the Bayesian approach, the administrator wisely allowed the opinions of the physicians who see the patients into the decision process. We have seen the havoc sampling error has raised with estimates.[5] It is possible that the sample estimate

---

[5] See chapter 1 the ten sample example.

obtained from the clinic would be very different from the true proportion of asthma patients. The opinions of the physicians have provided some anchor for the posterior estimate. By including the physician estimates, the administrator reaps the benefit of clinic physician experience and the sample estimate.

This does not yet commonly occur in large clinical trials. Because such a trial is designed using the frequentist approach, there is no way to formally incorporate the opinions of the many physicians who contribute their patients into its intellectual repository. These physician opinions we acknowledge as being by necessity biased. However, they provide useful information about the clinical event rate of interest and the efficacy of the intervention. Bayesian procedures admit the experiences of these physicians into the estimates of the vital parameters of the trial.

It is important to emphasize this point. A physician's biased opinion should not be rejected out of hand. Biased estimates can be good estimates, just as unbiased estimates can be bad estimates. As a simple example of this principle, consider the problem of computing the average cholesterol level of subjects in a cholesterol screening program for one day. Observer 1 decides to take the cholesterol level of each individual, and before taking the average, adds five mg/dl to each patient measurement. This is clearly a biased estimate. Observer 2 chooses to compute the usual average cholesterol, and then flip a coin. If its heads, he adds 50 mg/dl to the result. If it is tails, he subtracts 50 mg/dl. Observers 2's estimate of the average cholesterol is unbiased, while that of observer 1 is biased, but on any given day, we would be more comfortable with the biased estimate. In this example, the long-term behavior of the estimate is unhelpful.

Conclusion

The Bayesian approach to statistical analysis provides makes unique contributions. It explicitly considers prior distribution information. It allows construction of a loss function that directly and clearly states the loss (or gain) for each decision. It has admirable flexibility where traditional p values are murky, e.g., on the level of loss and community protection to be provided by the test.

However, Bayesian p values are not manna from heaven. The requirement of a specification of the prior distribution can be a burden if there is not much good information about the parameter to be estimated. What should that prior distribution be? What shape should it have? Should it be normally distributed, or follow some other distribution like a χ^2 distribution? What are the parameters of this distribution? This should be determined before any conclusions are drawn. Since the results will be based on this assumption, it is often useful to consider how the results change if the underlying prior distribution changes. Also, as we have seen with very simple prior distributions and familiar conditional distributions, computations for the posterior distribution can be problematic. Computing tools have eased this pain, but to the nonstatistician, the underlying mathematics can be intimidating. Similarly, a detailed loss function is required before the Bayesian action can be computed. Bayesian statistician's fret over this specification, while frequentists ignore it. Of course, retrospective Bayesian prior distributions and retrospective loss functions, chosen when the research program is over, are just as corruptive and just as worthless as retrospective alpha level thresholds.

Perhaps both the Bayes approach and the frequentist approach to statistical inference each should be viewed as mere tools in a toolkit. One should use the approach that fits the problem. If there is good prior information and high hopes of constructing a defensible loss function, it is difficult to argue against the Bayesian approach to statistical inference. However, if there is little or no prior information and no hope for consensus on a loss function, the worker might be best served by staying with the classical perspective. In any event, the worker must decide, and decide prospectively.

References

1. Berger, J.O., (1980) *Statistical Decision Theory. Foundations, Concepts and Methods.* Springer-Verlag, New York.
2. Lindley, D.V., (1976) "Inference for a Bernoulli process (a Bayesian view)", *The American Statistician* 30:112–118.
3. Pratt, J.W., (1962) "Discussion of A. Birnbaum's On the foundations of statistical inference," *Journal of the American Statistical Association* 57:269–326.

11

CHAPTER

Blind Guides for Explorers: *P* Values, Subgroups and Data Dredging

Unsuspected Pots of Gold

Research investigators are trained to be thorough, to find every-thing worth findings in their data. Having invested great time and effort in their studies, these scientists want and need to examine the data systematically and completely. In clinical experiments where there are multiple endpoints, investigators will examine the effect of therapy on each one, with the anticipated reward of identifying a therapy effect for the experiment's primary end-point. However, investigators are aware that there may be un-anticipated findings in other analyses, that, unlike the primary endpoint analysis, are nonprospectively stated evaluations. Inves-tigators believe that, like unsuspected pots of gold, these tantaliz-ing surprises might lie just under the surface, hidden from view, waiting to be found. If the experiment demonstrated that an in-tervention reduces the incidence of heart attacks, then maybe there is a hidden relationship between marital status and heart attacks. Perhaps there is an unanticipated relationship between the patient's astrologic sign and the occurrence of a heart attack? Sometimes it is not the investigator who is raising these questions. In the process of publication, reviewers of the manuscript will sometimes ask that additional analyses be carried out. These analyses can include considering the effect of the intervention in subsets of the data. Does the therapy work equally well in women

251

and men? Does it work equally in different racial groups? What about in patients with a previous heart attack? These analyses are demanded by others, but are also not prospectively stated.

The research program's cost-effectiveness and the desire for thoroughness require that all facets of a research effort's data be thoroughly examined. After all, why collect the data if it will not be considered in an analysis? However, as we have seen earlier,[1] the interpretation of nonprospective analyses is fraught with difficulty. The need to protect the community from the dissemination of mistaken results from research programs runs head-on into the need to make maximum use of the data so carefully collected. These problems are compounded when investigators begin to look at the findings in the experiment for just a subset (termed subgroup) of patients.

Confirmatory vs. Exploratory Analyses

The essential difference between confirmatory analyses and exploratory analyses is timing and planning. Confirmatory analyses are planned prospectively to insure that the appropriate data are precisely collected, and that bias-reducing protective mechanisms are in place. Type I error bounds for confirmatory analysis plans are provided and are set before the data are collected. A power analysis is completed to insure relationships between variables in the population are very likely to be embedded in the sample. Having the analysis plan in place before the data are collected insures that the findings in the data (which contains sampling error) do not influence the analysis plan.[2] The analysis for the primary endpoint is a confirmatory analysis. If the precepts in chapters 7 and 8 are followed, the analysis of secondary endpoints can be confirmatory as well.

Exploratory analysis, or in its worst form, data dredging, is the antithesis of confirmatory analysis. Exploratory analyses are often not prospectively announced. There is no a priori statement about type I error or type II error, therefore there is no clear

---

[1] The issue of interpretation of multiple endpoints was discussed in chapters 7 and 8.

[2] The issue of sampling error and its effect on analysis plans is discussed in chapter 1.

consideration of the implications for the scientific community of promulgating false and misleading results. While exploratory analysis may have some semblance of structure (e.g., looking for new baseline determinants of mortality in a clinical trial), according to James L. Miles [1], data dredging is the examination of all possible relationships in a database for significance.

Subgroup analysis is the examination of only a fraction of patients in a dataset. Every dataset includes different subcohorts. There are demographic subcohorts, subcohorts based on morbidity (e.g., patients who had hypertension or diabetes at the time of entry into the study). Subgroup analysis can either be confirmatory or reflect data dredging. What determines this characterization is (1) when the analysis was planned and (2) whether thoughtful type I and type II error issues have been considered a priori. For each subgroup, the effect of the intervention can be evaluated. Rarely is subgroup analysis included as a confirmatory analysis.[3]

Typically, after investigators have completed the limited number of confirmatory analyses that have been prospectively specified in the research program's protocol, the data dredging begins. If confirmatory analyses can be described as the process by which a selected well planned, circumscribed treasure site is excavated for a jewel that all reliable evidence suggests is present, then data dredging represents the complete and methodical strip mining of the site, churning up the information landscape, looking for any pattern at all in the data and proclaiming that the association leeched from the sample is present in the population. Data dredging and subgroup analyses are, by and large, unannounced, but they are almost always carried out. Conclusions from data dredging and subgroup analyses are often drawn as though every association in the sample reflects a true association in the population, i.e., as though there is no sampling error. "If you torture your data long enough, they will tell you whatever you want to hear," proclaims James Miles[1].

The problem with such an exhaustive examination is that the dataset contains many red herrings and false leads that are due to sampling error. In the process of selecting a dataset, sampling

---

[3] Two important counter examples are SHEP (Systolic Hypertension in the Elderly Program) and ALLHAT (Antihypertensive and Lipid Lowering Treatment to Prevent Heart Attack Trial) each of which make prospective statements for the subgroups to be analysed in the trial's conclusion. However, in neither case were prospective statements made concerning type I error for these subgroups.

error appears. The dataset will contain relationships that are embedded in the populations and relationships that are not. Such findings are misleading and can misdirect the scientific community. For example, from the MRFIT trial, the identification of a relationship that suggested that the treatment of hypertension may be harmful in men with abnormal hearts confused the medical community for several years[4]. In the end, this finding was attributed to sampling error. These spurious relationships appear because only a small number of subjects were chosen for the sample, and the pattern exists only for those subjects. If a greater number of subjects were selected, the pattern would disappear. The difficulty is that one cannot be certain when a pattern appearing in the sample is a true reflection of a pattern appearing in the population. We must keep in mind that a dataset's value is limited to the degree to which it accurately reflects the findings in the population.

The sample may also suggest that there is no relationship between variables when in fact the association does exist in the population. Relationships appearing in the population may not be apparent in the sample, again because of sampling error. How is the researcher to know which pattern in the sample is truly a pattern in the population and whether variables which are unrelated in the sample are in fact unrelated in the population?

Each Diminishes the Whole

Subgroup analysis refers to examining the findings of a research effort's endpoint(s) for only one of the many subsets of the entire cohort. There are many different subgroups in a trial. For each subgroup, the effect of the intervention can be evaluated and the interpretation of individual subgroup findings from a large clinical trial is a hazardous undertaking. The effect of the intervention for the entire cohort is divided among effects for many different subgroups. The practice of sound clinical trial methodology aids the evaluation of a well designed experiment's main, prospectively declared endpoint for the entire cohort of the trial. However, the well focused assessment of that intervention's effect for the prospectively designed endpoint is often blurred when the attention turns to subgroups. For each subgroup, a new p value is gen-

---

[4] See chapter 2.

erated, which cries for interpretation. Unfortunately, many of the important principles of good experimental methodology are missing in the direct examination of interesting subgroups. The choice of subgroups, inadequate sample size, low power, and the generation of multiple p values combine to create an environment in which the implications of therapy efficacy within the subgroups is diffuse and unclear.

The single most important tool the researcher has to protect herself against the hazard of data dredging is the a priori statement of (1) the associations she hopes to find and (2) what subgroups will be evaluated (3) what type I error she is willing to pay for drawing a conclusion about the association. Thereby, the research effort can be designed to minimize the number of database interrogations, minimizing the opportunities for sampling error to influence the findings. In the absence of these a priori statements, the best advice is that offered by Yusuf [2]—use the overall trial results to indicate the likely effect of the exposure or treatment in a particular subgroup.

Sampling error induces many relationships that are spurious. Consider a clinical trial designed to assess the role of LDL cholesterol level modification in reducing the incidence of the clinical endpoint fatal heart attack/nonfatal heart attack/revascularization. The analysis of the effect of therapy on this endpoint in the entire cohort was overwhelming positive. The examination of this effect across several subgroups are provided in Table 11.1.

Table 11.1 reveals the effect of therapy within each of six subgroups (A through F) in the clinical trial. None of these analyses was announced a priori. Each subgroup contains two different strata. For each stratum, the number of patients in the subgroup at risk of getting the endpoint, who have the endpoint, and the cumulative incidence rate is provided. To assess the effect of therapy, both the relative risk of therapy and the p value are included. For example, in subgroup A we have two strata I and II. In strata I there are 576 patients; 126 of them experienced the endpoint. The cumulative incidence of the endpoint in the placebo group was 27.59 (i.e., 27.59 percent of these patients experienced a clinical endpoint); in the active group this was 16.08. The relative risk due to therapy was 0.54, i.e., the risk of an event in the active group was 54 percent of the risk of that event in the placebo group, suggesting that there was some benefit was associated with therapy. The p value for this protective effect was 0.001. In this subgroup, the effect of therapy was notable in each

Table 11.1. Effect of therapy on endpoint incidence within blinded subgroups Fatal and nonfatal MI plus revascularizations

	Subgroup	Patients			P-Value	Rel Risk
		Placebo	Active	Total		
A	I					
	Endpoint	80	46	126		
	Total	290	286	576		
	Cum. Inc Rate *100	27.59	16.08	21.88	0.001	0.54
	II					
	Endpoint	469	384	853		
	Total	1788	1795	3583		
	Cum. Inc Rate *100	26.23	21.39	23.81	0.001	0.80
B	I					
	Endpoint	258	217	475		
	Total	1003	1027	2030		
	Cum. Inc Rate *100	25.72	21.13	23.40	0.018	0.80
	II					
	Endpoint	291	213	504		
	Total	1075	1054	2129		
	Cum. Inc Rate *100	27.07	20.21	23.67	<0.001	0.73
C	I					
	Endpoint	98	95	193		
	Total	461	439	900		
	Cum. Inc Rate *100	21.26	21.64	21.44	0.916	1.02
	II					
	Endpoint	451	335	786		
	Total	1617	1642	3259		
	Cum. Inc Rate *100	27.89	20.40	24.12	<0.001	0.71
D	I					
	Endpoint	105	91	196		
	Total	397	402	799		
	Cum. Inc Rate *100	26.45	22.64	24.53	0.210	0.84
	II					
	Endpoint	444	339	783		
	Total	1681	1679	3360		
	Cum. Inc Rate *100	26.41	20.19	23.30	<0.001	0.75
E	I					
	Endpoint	186	137	323		
	Total	653	639	1292		
	Cum. Inc Rate *100	28.48	21.44	25.00	0.011	0.75

Table 11.1 (*cont.*)

	Subgroup	Patients				Rel
		Placebo	Active	Total	P-Value	Risk
	II					
	Endpoint	363	293	656		
	Total	1425	1442	2867		
	Cum. Inc Rate *100	25.47	20.32	22.88	0.001	0.77
F	I					
	Endpoint	214	165	379		
	Total	802	833	1635		
	Cum. Inc Rate *100	26.68	19.81	23.18	0.002	0.73
	II					
	Endpoint	335	265	600		
	Total	1276	1248	2524		
	Cum. Inc Rate *100	26.25	21.23	23.77	0.004	0.79

of the two strata, (relative risk of 0.54 in stratum I vs. 0.80 in strata II) with a further suggestion that patients in strata I received a greater benefit from therapy than patients in stratum II.

The finding of uniform therapy effect across the strata does not hold for each of the six subgroups. For some of these subgroups, the effect of therapy was quite reduced in one of the two strata. In subgroup C, for example, the relative risk for the event is 1.02 (p value = 0.916) for strata I, suggesting no benefit. In stratum II for this subgroup, the relative risk is 0.71 (*p* value <0.001). Does this suggest that patients in subgroup C, strata I should not receive the therapy? If true, this would be an important message to disseminate, especially if the therapy was associated with significant cost or side effects. There is a similar finding for subgroup D, in which, again, stratum I demonstrates no effect of therapy while strata II demonstrates a possibly important effect. Subgroup E suggests that in each of its two strata, the effect of therapy is the same. Subgroups B and F each suggest that there may be a stratum dependent therapy effect.

The point of this exercise is that we do not know how to integrate sampling error into this equation. We cannot see which results are spurious and which ones reflect true relationships in the population based on the effect sizes and *p* values. We cannot just look at the *p* values to help us decide because of the accumulation of Type I error associated with multiple *p* value (here there are twelve p values) interpretations. With each new p values we increase the background noise, decreasing our ability to hear the signal. There are too many of them.

Adding in the identities of the subgroups and their strata provides interesting perspective. But how much new information is there?

Table 11.2 contains the same subgroup data analysis as did table 11.1, but this time the subgroup identities are added. Subgroups A (gender), B (age) and C (baseline LDL cholesterol) provides examination of scientific interest. Subgroups D, E, and F do not. Each of these last three subgroups represent merely a random grouping of the data. From a comparison of Table 11.1 and 11.2, we see that one cannot differentiate a meaningful effect of therapy from just the random play of chance.

Even if we concentrate on the first three subgroups whose subgroup definitions are plausible and have scientific meaning, we still cannot be sure that the effects demonstrated in Table 11.2 truly represent the findings in the population. The gender examination suggests that women derive a greater benefit from cholesterol reduction therapy then do men. There appears to be no real difference in effect of therapy across the different age strata. And, it appears that patients with baseline LDL cholesterol greater than 125 mg/dl derived a profound effect from therapy while those patients with a baseline LDL cholesterol ≤ 125 mg/dl obtain no benefit from therapy.

These findings for women and for patients with baseline LDL cholesterol ≤ 125 mg/dl were obtained from the CARE clinical trial and published by Sacks et al [5], producing much discussion among lipidologists. A follow-up manuscript elaborating on the effect of cholesterol reduction therapy in women was published by Lewis et al [6]. A manuscript examining the relationship between LDL cholesterol and clinical endpoints was also published in 1998[7]. The subgroup findings from CARE and the subsequent published manuscripts based on these findings were surprising and useful, generating much debate. In neither case was the hypothesis stated prospectively (with alpha allocation) in the protocol.[5] Yet, in each case the subgroup analysis was relevant and insisted upon by the scientific community. How can one interpret the findings of these required but non-prospective evaluations?

---

[5] The propsectively written plan which outlines the goal, design, execution, and analysis of the experiment.

Table 11.2. Effect of therapy endpoint incidence within blinded subgroups Fatal and nonfatal MI plus revascularizations

	Subgroup	Patients Placebo	Active	Total	P-Value	Rel Risk
Gender	Male					
A	Endpoint	80	46	126		
	Total	290	286	576		
	Cum. Inc Rate *100	27.59	16.08	21.88	0.001	0.54
	Female					
	Endpoint	469	384	853		
	Total	1788	1795	3583		
	Cum. Inc Rate *100	26.23	21.39	23.81	0.001	0.80
Age	≤59					
B	Endpoint	258	217	475		
	Total	1003	1027	2030		
	Cum. Inc Rate *100	25.72	21.13	23.40	0.018	0.80
	>59					
	Endpoint	291	213	504		
	Total	1075	1054	2129		
	Cum. Inc Rate *100	27.07	20.21	23.67	<0.001	0.73
LDL	≤125 mg/dl					
Cholesterol	Endpoint	98	95	193		
C	Total	461	439	900		
	Cum. Inc Rate *100	21.26	21.64	21.44	0.916	1.02
	>125 mg/dl					
	Endpoint	451	335	786		
	Total	1617	1642	3259		
	Cum. Inc Rate *100	27.89	20.40	24.12	<0.001	0.71
Random	I					
D	Endpoint	105	91	196		
	Total	397	402	799		
	Cum. Inc Rate *100	26.45	22.64	24.53	0.210	0.84
	II					
	Endpoint	444	339	783		
	Total	1681	1679	3360		
	Cum. Inc Rate *100	26.41	20.19	23.30	<0.001	0.75
Random	I					
E	Endpoint	186	137	323		
	Total	653	639	1292		
	Cum. Inc Rate *100	28.48	21.44	25.00	0.011	0.75

Table 11.2 (*cont.*)

	Subgroup	Patients Placebo	Active	Total	P-Value	Rel Risk
	II					
	Endpoint	363	293	656		
	Total	1425	1442	2867		
	Cum. Inc Rate *100	25.47	20.32	22.88	0.001	0.77
Random	I					
F	Endpoint	214	165	379		
	Total	802	833	1635		
	Cum. Inc Rate *100	26.68	19.81	23.18	0.002	0.73
	II					
	Endpoint	335	265	600		
	Total	1276	1248	2524		
	Cum. Inc Rate *100	26.25	21.23	23.77	0.004	0.79

One relevant tool for assessing subgroup results is the criterion of confirmation or replication of an experiment's results. In its narrowest form, study replication involves the slavish reproduction of previous numeric results using the original experimental protocol; its goal is to limit investigator error (either inadvertent or intentional) [8]. More broadly, replication involves the systematic variation of research conditions to determine whether an earlier result can be observed under new conditions. This is particularly important when a number of different study designs are used. The variety of study designs, each with its own unique strengths and weaknesses, minimizes the chance that all of the studies are making the same mistake. Consistency is demonstrated by several of these studies giving the same results [9].

It is this broader, more useful interpretation that would be most helpful in interpreting the results from CARE. An independent clinical trial carried out in Australia [10], completed after the end of CARE, examined the effect of the same cholesterol reducing therapy. This second study was different from CARE in that (1) the Australian study (known by the acronym LIPID) was twice as large as CARE, (2) the entry criteria were somewhat different, and (3) the clinical endpoint LIPID was coronary heart disease death, a more reliable endpoint than the well-accepted combined endpoint of fatal heart attack/nonfatal heart attack/revascularization used in the CARE subgroup analysis. The LIPID investigators carried out the subgroup analyses in women and in patients with low levels of baseline LDL cholesterol. They found no differential effect of therapy in women, a finding that contradicted the observation of CARE. However, the Australian study did replicate the baseline LDL cholesterol subgroup findings first identified in CARE. Thus, one would give more credence to the replicated finding involving baseline LDL cholesterol than to the finding involving women. The lesson is that subgroup analyses from one study are difficult to interpret on their own. They should be reproduced in an independent study before they are considered reliable.

How to Interpret Exploratory Analyses

It is easy to bash exploratory analyses after the above demonstration; one certainly cannot blur the implication of hypothesis testing (i.e., confirmatory) analyses with the results of hypothesis generating efforts. However, hypothesis generating efforts should not be relegated to second-class (or no-class) research. Exploratory analyses play a useful, vital role in the advance of medicine. Ideas for breakthrough therapy more often than not have their basis in discerning examination of data already in place. Astute observations in concert with deductive reasoning have always and should always play an important role in investigational efforts.

Therefore, a hypothesis generating research effort should not consist of a sloppy, lackadaisical, second-class evaluation "just because it is exploratory." Exploratory research should not be synonymous with haphazard or poorly executed work. A good exploratory analysis should first be accurately described for what it is. The manuscript should state that the analyses are post hoc and retrospective. The exploration should be carefully considered, with the regions of the exploration well mapped. The analysis tool should also be determined before the data interrogation begins.

The definition of subgroups in clinical trials is critical. Yusuf [4] states that all subgroups be proper subgroups, i.e., that the criteria for patient inclusion of subgroups be determined at baseline. This avoids the difficulty of attributing differences at the trial's end to subgroup definition. Since no follow-up event can influence a patient's subgroup membership, the subgroup's character is not affected by events occurring after baseline that are related to the effect of therapy.

As we have seen, p values have become a common tool for the evaluation of treatment effects. However they are of dubious value in an examination that is not prospectively formulated and for which the experiment was not designed. This is precisely the situation with subgroup analysis. In addition, the construction of a subgroup evaluation does not permit balancing the assignment of active vs. control therapy within each subgroup strata through randomization. This resulting imbalance clouds the interpretation of p values because the effect they identify may not be fully attributable to the therapy. In addition, the issue of what to do with multiple p values requires careful thought. Even with the liberal assumption that the multiple post hoc hypothesis tests are independent of one another, the maximum acceptable Type I error for each test must be uselessly small in order to control the overall probability of making at least one type I error in the entire analysis.[6] The realization that the tests are not independent because the same patient occurs in more than one subgroup clouds the interpretation of p values further.

Interpreting subgroup analyses is like trying to find your way through uncharted back country. The last thing you need is a blind guide, and that is precisely what nominal, un-prespecified p values are. When readers see p values listed by the tens or by the hundreds in a published manuscript or presentation, the temptation is sometimes overwhelming to rank order than, perhaps unconsciously relating the small p values to larger effects. But, as we saw in chapter 5, small p values do not indicate large effect sizes[7]. Thus the rank ordering conveys little about which effects are "more important" than others. Consideration of the total alpha error expended[8] complicates the use of p values in this setting, probably beyond recognition.

Exploratory analyses do not draw conclusions. They are designed not to confirm results and promulgate findings to be put

---

[6] This would not be an issue if prospective thought was given to alpha expenditure (see Chapters 7 and 8).

[7] For example, a very large sample size can portray a clinically small effect with a small p value.

[8] Discussed in chapter 8.

into place in the community, but to instead provide a sense of what the findings might be; they lay the framework for additional confirmatory work. A manuscript based on an exploratory analysis would be truer to its research nature if p values were not reported. Reporting z scores conveys the size of the effect size after correcting for (dividing by) its standard error. Reporting Z scores rather than p values clearly conveys the sense that no hypothesis testing is underway. In exploratory analysis, the goal is hypothesis generation, and not hypothesis confirmation. With no ability to generalize their results, exploratory analyses are not helped by p values.

Power must also be provided to aid in the interpretation of the reported risk reductions for the presented subgroup analyses. Power is much like a searchlight; before we can believe that the search for a therapy effect in a subgroup is negative, we must be assured that the light was bright enough to find the effect. If a subgroup analysis contains subminimal power (power <80 percent), the evaluation of the effect size of these groups is particularly hazardous. This choice of a suboptimal power level is an attempt at compromise. Although maximum power is desirable in subgroup evaluation, it is often logistically and financially impossible to attain. As pointed out by Yusef et. al. [4], the expense of clinical trials restricts them to only the sample size required for the minimum power acceptable to test the hypothesis in the entire randomized cohort. Subgroups will not provide the number of patients required to test the trial hypothesis. This was true in SAVE (Survival and Ventricular Enlargement) [11,12]. SAVE was designed to test the effect of anitconverting enzyme inhibitor (ACEi) therapy on mortality in patients with left ventricular dysfunction after a heart attack. The total SAVE cohort size of 2231 did not allow for adequate numbers of patients within the subgroups to provide optimal power. However, a priori acknowledgement that power in subgroups will be less than in the minimal acceptable power for the trial's entire cohort is not sufficient reason to discard the notion of using power in interpretation of subgroup data. A use of a new minimal power level as a guideline in interpreting the subgroup data from these trials may hold promise. This analysis in SAVE demonstrated that, in subgroups with at least 50% power the point estimates were all supportive of a captopril benefit for total mortality and cardiovascular mortality/morbidity [13].

Caveat emptor: Let the Buyer Beware.

Knowledge that the manuscript in one's hand is primarily hypothesis generating does not give the reader the right to turn a blind eye to it. Hypothesis generation work should be considered the first databased view of the future of the research issue. A first reconnaissance, though not always optimal, is almost always suggestive of future findings. However, the key to interpreting subgroup analysis and ferreting out data dredging is care and vigilance. Exploratory studies should provide complete disclosure about how many analyses were carried out, not just the ones reported. Good exploratory analyses will not treat every positive result as a confirmed a major hypothesis. As J.L. Miles [1] states "If the fishing expedition catches a boot, the fishermen should throw it back, not claim that they were fishing for boots." There should be a clear biologically plausible mechanism motivating the subgroup analysis to make it persuasive. Consider the tenets of causality[9] as criteria for assessing subgroup results. If a finding was prospectively specified, contains adequate community level protection (type I and type II errors are low), has no temporal ambiguity between variables and has analogous findings from other studies, it is more likely than not to reflect a true finding in the population.

Conclusions

Data dredging is a search for significance, and the dredgers are driven by the notion that if they look hard enough, long enough, and dig deep enough they will turn up something "significant." While it is possible to turn up a jewel in this strip mining operation, for every rare jewel identified, there will be many false finds, fakes, and shams. It takes tremendous effort to sort these findings all out, and we are reminded of the warning from James Johnson. In his book *Experimental Agriculture* (1849),[10] Johnson stated that a badly conceived experiment not only wasted time and money, but led to the adoption of incorrect results into stan-

---

[9] The useful criteria developed by epidemiologists in assessing whether an association between variables is a causal one.
[10] Discussed in Chapter 1.

dard books, the loss of money in practice, and to the neglect of further research.

Exploratory research efforts can shed first light on new directions for future research, but they must not masquerade as confirmatory analyses. An exploratory analysis can be of great value if it is announced prospectively, exerts discipline through the early choice of an analysis plan, and limits itself to examinations that are plausible based on the understanding of the mechanism of the disease. In choosing subgroups, the investigator needs to insure that there is some balance in the subgroups by therapy, especially if the number of subjects in each subgroup is small. In addition, subgroup analyses should be accompanied by an assessment of power.

Finally p values should be avoided in exploratory analyses. P values measure the role of sampling error in research results as one considers whether the findings should be generalized to the community. Exploratory analyses can make no such generalization, since the analysis is itself data driven and type I error cannot be accurately computed. The many significance tests generated from nonprospective exploratory analyses only serve to tighten the covers over the eyes of these blind guides.

References

1. Mills, J.L. (1993) "Data torturing," *New Eng J Med.* 329:1196–1199.
2. The SHEP Cooperative Research Group. (1988) "Rationale and design of a randomized clinical trial on prevention of stroke in isolated systolic hypertension," *Journal of Clinical Epidemiology* 41:1197–1208.
3. Davis, B.R., Cutler, J.A., Gordon, D.J., Furberg, C.D., Wright, J.T., Cushman,C., Grimm, R.H., LaRosa, J., Whelton, P.K., Perry, H.M., Alderman, M.H., Ford, C.E., Oparil, S., Francis, C., Proscham, M., Pressel, S., Black, H.R., and Hawkins, C.M., for the ALLHAT Research Group. (1996) "Rationale and design for the antihypertensive and lipid lowering treatment to prevent heart attack trial," *American Journal of Hypertension* 9:342–360.
4. Yusef, S., Wittes, J., Probstfield, J., and Tyroler, H.A., (1991) "Analysis and Interpretation of Treament Effects in Subgroups of Patients in Randomized Clinical Trials," *Journal of the American Medical Association* 2266:93–98.
5. Sacks, F.M., Pfeffer, M.A., Moyé, L.A., Rouleau, J.L., Rutherford, J.D., Cole, T.G., Brown, L., Warnica, J.W., Arnold, J.M., Wun, C.C.,

Davis, B.R., and Braunwald, E., for the Cholesterol and recurrent Events Trial Investigators (1996) "The effect of pravastatin on coronary events after myocardial infarction in patients with average cholesterol levels," *N Engl J Med* 335:1001–1009.

6. Lewis, S.J., Sacks, F.M., Mitchell, J.S., East, C., Glasser, S., Kell, S., Letterer, R., Limacher, M., Moyé, L.A., Rouleau, J.L., Pfeffer, M.A., and Braunwald, E., (1998) "Effect of pravastatin on cardiovascular events in women after myocardial infarction: the cholesterol and recurrent events (CARE) trial," *Journal of the American College of Cardiology* 32:140–146.

7. Sacks, F.M., Moyé, L.A., Davis, B.R., Cole, T.G., Rouleau, J.L., Nash, D.T., Pfeffer, M.A., and Braunwald, E. (1998) "Relationship between plasma LDL concentrations during treatment with pravastatin and recurrent coronary events in the Cholesterol and Recurrent Events trial," *Circulation* 97:1446–1452.

8. Cohen, A.J. "Replication" *Epidemiology* 8:341–343.

9. Beaglehole, R., Bonita, R. and Kjellström, T., (1993) *Causation in epidemiology*, Geneva: World Health Organization, pp. 71–81.

10. The Long-Term Intervention with Pravastatin in Ischaemic Disease (LIPID) Study Group. (1998) "Prevention of cardiovascular events and death with pravastatin in patients with coronary heart disease with a broad range of initial cholesterol levels," *New Eng J Med* 339:1349–57.

11. Moyé, L.A., for the SAVE Cooperative Group (1991) "Rationale and Design of a Trial to Assess Patient Survival and Ventricular Enlargement after Myocardial Infarction," *Journal of the American College of Cardiology*, 68:70D–79D.

12. Pfeffer, M.A., Brauwald, E., and Moyé L.A., (1992) "Effect of Captopril on mortality and morbidity in patients with left ventricular dysfunction after myocardial infarction—results of the Survival and Ventricular Enlargement Trial," *New England Journal of Medicine* 327:669–677.

13. Moyé, L.A., Pfeffer, M.A., Wun, C.C., and Davis, B.R., (1994) "Uniformity of Captopril Benefit in the Post Infarction Population: Subgroup Analysis in SAVE," *European Heart Journal* 15:2–8.

Conclusions: Good Servants but Bad Masters

Researchers who ignore sampling error's impact while drawing conclusions from sample based research are like pilots who ignore gravity's impact while flying an aircraft. P values help us determine the influence of sampling error on the conclusion we draw from research programs, by encapsulating the sampling errors contained in the research's data. However, that is all that they do. P values have risen to an unjustified role of preeminence in medical research. Bradford Hill (speaking of the chi square test) described them as good servants, but bad masters. That is a lesson in health care research that we must still learn. By ceding our best judgment to their rule, must is lost.

For ethical, fiscal, logistical and administrative reasons, the researchers can only study a tiny fraction of the targeted patients. The researchers are extremely interested in extending the results from the sample to the population. Essentially the extension requires taking the findings from the small sample that the researchers studied, observed, and carefully documented, and then apply these findings to thousands (and often millions) of patients who have not been directly observed and studied. There is no doubt that extension is both a necessary and a hazardous process. It is made more dangerous by the recognition that several competent researchers can each independently evaluate different samples from the same population. Since the samples are different, the sample results they wish to extend to the population are different. As we have seen all to often, this cacophony of conflicting scientific results leads to chaos and policy gridlock.

The scientific community has developed a collection of guidelines which when followed, allow the safest extension of the small sample findings to the larger population. These guidelines are simple. First, establish a procedure by which research is peer-reviewed, i.e. carefully scrutinized and criticized by a small number of experts. These results appear in peer-reviewed medical and scientific journals. This is a sign that the study's methodology is consistent with the standard research procedures accepted by the scientific community. These articles must be given a greater priority than publications in non-peer-reviewed journals. Peer-reviewed journals are also superior to abstracts, which are only brief, preliminary reports of non-peer-reviewed work. Like houses built on shifting sands, contentions based on abstracts are unstable and unreliable. There are many examples of abstracts misdirecting medical thought, which was finally corrected by the appearance of the peer reviewed manuscript[1]. Abstracts, like the telephone call that sets up a blind date, promise much, but are often bitterly disappointing when the full view (of the data) finally becomes available.

Secondly, the ability to extend a research question's answer from a sample to a population depends on whether the research was designed to answer the question. Some research findings in the sample occur through "the freak of chance". The fisherman is suspect who returns from a fishing trip not with fish but with boots and claims that he was "fishing for boots all along". So too is the researcher who claims he has an important answer from his sample when he never intended to ask that research question of his sample. He just happened to find it in the sample. This is an important problem in research interpretation given the tendency among many researchers and their advocates to "analyze everything, and report what is favorable to our belief". This regrettably unstructured tendency chokes the research information stream by mixing in with the few, good prospectively asked research questions many ancillary analyses addressing research questions which were not asked prospectively. The research team does not plan these additional analyses when they are designing their ex-

---

[1] Best example of being misled by an abstract is that of Weissman, in which the subsequent peer-reviewed publication contradicted the first preliminary findings announced in the abstract.

periment. They contain many red herrings and false leads. These ancillary analyses are instead "tacked on" during the experiment or at the end of the experiment after everyone has seen what the data show.

The established way to avoid this difficult problem is to insist that research results be provided at two levels.[2] The highest level is occupied by those questions asked by the investigator before any data were obtained. These questions are often small in number, well considered, and, more specifically, had the research design sculptured to provide answers to them. The maxim "first say what you plan to do, then do what you say" leads to the clearest extension of the research's results from the small sample to the large population. The second tier questions are merely exploratory questions, or hypothesis generating questions. The definitive answers provided to this second group of questions must wait until the next research effort, because the research that spawned them was not designed to answer them.

Subgroup analysis falls into this second tier, or exploratory analysis for very simple reasons. First, sometimes it is difficult to identify whether a patient falls into a subgroup or not unless some prospective criteria are defined (for example does duration of exposure mean continuous exposure or intermittent exposure); the determination is clearest if the definition is made up front. In addition, since subgroups are only part of the sample (for example only males, or only Hispanics), the number of patients in the subgroup can be small. The total sample itself is typically barely large enough to justify extending results to the population at large. Subgroup analysis reduces the number of subjects even further. One can imagine taking a subgroup of only Hispanics, then only Hispanic males, then only Hispanic males <45 years old, then Hispanic males <45 years old with weight >200 lbs. The subgroup gets smaller and smaller, with each "cut" making the extension of the risk factor—disease association to the population even more hazardous. The extensions of findings from a sample to the population are hazardous enough without trying to extend the findings of smaller subgroups. Subgroup analyses, like "fool's gold" should be viewed with a jaundiced and skeptical eye, and not be accepted without independent confirmation from a second study. Thus the research question must be asked prospectively (the fisherman

---

[2] Refer to Chapters 1 and 11.

must declare what he is fishing for before he shoves off) and based on a fixed analysis plan which analyses random data.

I have placed a great emphasis on the prospective nature of research for two reasons. The first involves the notion of the sample. Since a sample examines only a fraction of the population, it may contain relationships that are not in the population, or the population may contain a relationship that is not in the sample. With every decision we make about a relationship in the sample, we run the risk of drawing a mistaken inference about the relationship in the population. The community pays a real price for these types of error, as ineffective care are inflicted on them or they are denied effective care due to underpowered experiments. To minimize these errors, we keep track of p values and power.

But, as important as p values are for measuring sampling error, we are reminded that that is all that they do. P values are not the sole source of judgment for the study. They do not measure effect size, nor do they convey the extent of study discordance. A small p value does not in and of itself mean that the sample size is adequate, that the effect size is clinically meaningful, or that there is clear attribution of effect to the exposure or intervention of interest. These other factors must themselves be individually considered by a careful critical review of the research effort. Reflexively responding to p values is shortsighted thought evasion. We must examine each of these other important issues separately to gain a clear view of what the sample is saying about the population.

Other influences can distort our viewing lens as well. Through the wrong choice of dosage or poor choice of the population the research program may not be responsive to the question asked by the scientific community. Small p values cannot rescue poorly designed studies. High p values can reflect the inadequate power of the experiment, or the incorrect choice of exposure level. More commonly, however, well designed clinical trials are undermined by poor execution. Concordantly executed trials (i.e., executed according to the prospectively specified protocol) allow the cleanest and clearest interpretation of p values, while discordant trials (i.e., those that undergo a midcourse change in analysis plan or endpoint) can be impossible to interpret. Because the findings are so difficult for us to integrate into our fund of knowledge, these latter experiments are frustrating, ultimately representing a squandering of precious resources. Blurring the interpretation of p values through study discordance makes the view of the population through the sample unusable and the study a failure.

The alpha error levels required to decide against the null hypothesis are under the complete control of the investigators and require careful deliberate thought. These levels should not be ceded to a guideline unless it represents a well founded standard, and not just a historical tradition. I have provided several strategies that produce conservative, tightly controlled alpha and lead to clear interpretation of a concordantly executed, multi-armed, clinical trial with multiple endpoints. These strategies allow the investigator to choose a level of type I error symmetrically or asymmetrically. They are not the only strategies to choose from, and of course no investigator should be compelled to use them. However, investigators should choose something. They should be plain about their choice, stick to with their choice, and report the results of their choice. Readers of clinical trials should insist on this.

Physician investigators cannot understand alpha error concepts unless they understand the sampling error principles. Statisticians cannot provide the best advice on experimental design unless they understand the medical framework and underlying theory of the intervention or exposure. Statisticians and physician investigators must understand each other, investing the time and effort to communicate effectively, learning to appreciate the nuances of each other's language. Liking each other is preferable—understanding each other is essential.

Whether I believe in the p values of other researchers depends on their methodologic discipline. If they put great effort into the design of their research, building in a clear effect attribution, allocating alpha prospectively and ethically, and carry out the research concordantly, then I am able to integrate their p values with their effect sizes, precision, and sample size to come to a conclusion. However, if the research is not well designed and/or experiences severe discordancies in its execution, its p values must be rebuffed.

We physicians must control our inclination to explain any research result we read in a manuscript or hear from a lecturer. Ask first if these results are due to sampling error. If they are, we need not go forward with interesting theories about the research findings, and our time could be better placed elsewhere. Community protection is paramount. Even with adequate precautions, sampling error can still result in the wrong conclusion. Since the written and visual media quickly pass on new research findings for consumption by an increasingly health-conscious community, there is even less room and time for error. We should uphold community health by insuring that we do not expose it to the corrosive influences of misleading results. By standing now for community protection we can help to shape the future rather than be stampeded into it by sampling error.

I am often asked for rules or guidelines for interpreting medical research—the best rule I can give is this: use your head! Correct interpretation of a complicated experiment should never as simple as reading from a rulebook. We must carefully sift information about the state of health care in the community, the prospective nature of the research design, its concordant execution, and the appropriateness of the analysis plan before we can make decisions. Drawing conclusions for a community based on a sample of data is a thinking person's business. Of course, as we think we will make mistakes, but it has been my thesis that we are worse off if we let p values do our thinking for us. Nevertheless, in my view there are three important principles of research.They are simple, and, by and large, nonmathematical.

Lesson 1:   Provide for the general welfare of your patients.

This should not be reduced to the status of a truism. Patients volunteer their time their energy, and quite frankly, their health for taking part in the studies that researchers design and execute. Researchers are honor bound and obligated to insure that the participants in their studies receive the best available treatment. They are a precious resource never to be taken for granted and never to be squandered.

I have pointed out several areas where the ethics and the mathematics of clinical experiments collide, but this is not one of them. Consider for example, a four thousand patient clinical trial, designed to test the effect of therapy to reduce total mortality. If we assume the placebo event rate is 20%, then we expect $(2000)(0.20) = 400$ deaths in the placebo group. If we anticipate that the cumulative mortality rate in the treatment group is 0.16, we would expect $(2000)(0.16) = 320$ patients. Out of the four thousand patient trial, the entire measure of therapy effectiveness is reduced to the different experiences of $400 - 320 = 80$ patients. Clearly, if the investigators knew who these eighty patients were at the trial's inception, these patients would be singled out for very special care. Of course the investigator does not know the identities of these eighty patients. Therefore the investigator must treat *every* patient in the study like *that* patient is *the* patient that will make the difference in the trial.

Lesson 2:   Promote collegial relationships with your co-investigators.

Issues of publication policy, doses of medication, the characteristics of the patients to be included in the study are critical, and strong willed scientists can vehemently disagree on these fundamental trial characteristics. Investigators should expect this. However, they must actively work to insure that the communication between investigators does not become choked with anger, resentment or hostility, for if this is permitted to occur, the research effort is weakened and its survival threatened. Each investigator makes a unique contribution of personality, intellect and perspective, and deserves full expression and consideration. Investigators must remember that their quiet answers to wrathful questions from their strongly opinionated colleagues can blunt this anger, turning it aside. Research efforts undergo external, centrifugal forces (e.g., opposing points of view in the medical community, politically charged scientific issues, contrary findings in other research programs) which threaten to tear the resesarch effort apart. These destructive forces are counterbalanced by the centripetal force of investigators who are able to put their differences of opinion aside and hold their common effort together.

Lesson 3:   Preserve, protect and defend type I error.

Prospective statements of the questions to be answered by the research effort, and avoidance of data based changes in the protocol preserve the best measure of type I error, while simultaneously protecting patient communities from exposure to harmful placebos. By following the enunciated principles of this book, investigators will be able to recognize the menace of type I error to both the patient and scientific communities, control it, and report it. Adjustments to type I error are unavoidable. However, we must be ever vigilant to avoid the alpha corrupting influence of having the data determine the analysis plan.

Following these principles promotes a successful research program, that is, the construction and protection of a research enviornment that permits an objective assessment of the therapy or exposure being studied. If there is any fixed star in the research constellation, it is that sample based research must be hypothesis driven and concordantly executed to have real meaning for both the scientific community and the patient populations we serve.

Index